Clinical Leadership
for Paramedics

Clinical Leadership for Paramedics

Edited by Amanda Y. Blaber and Graham Harris

McGraw Hill Education Open University Press

Open University Press
McGraw-Hill Education
McGraw-Hill House
Shoppenhangers Road
Maidenhead
Berkshire
England
SL6 2QL

email: enquiries@openup.co.uk
world wide web: www.openup.co.uk

and Two Penn Plaza, New York, NY 10121-2289, USA

First published 2014

A catalogue record of this book is available from the British Library

ISBN-13: 978-0-335-26312-7
ISBN-10: 0-335-26312-7
eISBN: 978-0-335-26313-4

Library of Congress Cataloging-in-Publication Data
CIP data applied for

Typeset by Aptara Inc., India
Printed and bound by CPI Group (UK) Ltd, Croydon, CR0 4YY

Contents

List of figures

List of tables

Contributors

Amanda Blaber has worked at several universities offering various academic levels of paramedic study. Amanda currently works at the University of Brighton. Her clinical background is in Emergency Care. Amanda is very interested in the NHS as an organization and how culture within organizations has the potential to affect the overall approach to care and subsequently the quality of care. Organizations also have an effect on their employees, in terms of motivation, team-working and well-being. Amanda is Editor of the bestselling book *Foundations for Paramedic Practice*, 2nd edition, published by Open University Press in 2012, and co-edited *Assessment Skills for Paramedics* with Graham Harris, published by Open University Press in 2011.

Kevin Barrett has been Course Leader for the BSc (Hons) Paramedic Practice course at the University of Brighton since 2009. His clinical background is in intensive care nursing. Kevin recognizes the pivotal role that mentorship has in supporting students in challenging and demanding practice environments and, especially, the centrality of mentors' influence on students' development as clinicians.

Graham Harris, MSc, BSc, PGCE, Chartered MCIPD, MCPara, is a Senior Lecturer and Programme Leader – Professional Lead for the FdSc and BSc Paramedic Science programmes at the University of Greenwich. His clinical background is as a paramedic with nearly 40 years experience, including periods in the military, the NHS and academic arena. He is the College of Paramedics Director of Professional Standards, and the elected College's Governing Council member for London Region. He is also a Health and Care Professions Council Partner Visitor. He is committed to the development of the paramedic profession and the professional body. Graham is co-Editor of *Assessment Skills for Paramedics* with Amanda Blaber, which was published by Open University Press in 2011.

Paul Jones is a Senior Lecturer in Paramedic Practice at Liverpool John Moores University (LJMU). Paul's role takes him beyond practice and allows him to consider the art and science of being a modern paramedic. He leads the programme for the CPD Diploma, is an external examiner for another higher education (HE) institution and a bank paramedic with the North West Ambulance Service. Paul's current roles are a culmination of operational and educational experiences ranging from being an ambulance care assistant to being a training officer, and having a basic education before studying at varying Higher Education levels, finally achieving his Master's Degree in Research. LJMU has been delivering paramedic programmes since the transfer of education to HE, and continues to develop its capability to transfer knowledge. Leadership is core to all paramedic programmes – recognizing a personal characteristic is essential for good leaders and making decisions maintains their credibility. It is for these reasons that Paul has chosen to write the leadership and decision-making chapters within this text.

Linda Nelson, Med, PG (Dip), BSc (Hons), Diploma Nursing, RGN, is a Principal Lecturer, School of Health & Social Care, Teesside University. Linda is a qualified registered nurse and spent her professional career in practice working in critical care areas, including intensive care, coronary care and accident and emergency. She has worked in Higher Education for 13 years and is the subject leader for a large team of people who deliver education at all academic levels in specialist subjects, including paramedic science and nursing. Effective leadership skills are fundamental to the success of this role and utilized on a daily basis. Linda has been actively involved in the development of paramedic education at Teesside and its success has required close partnership working with both North East and Yorkshire Ambulance services. Linda has a strong interest in preceptorship and was seconded to North East Ambulance Service as a project lead to implement the concept in the Trust.

Mel Newton, as an experienced Registered Nurse, gained substantial leadership and management expertise within her clinical role after qualifying in 1985 till 2001 when she managed care services for older adults. Mel's clinical experience was within an Acute Trust environment as well as a community setting. Mel began her Higher Education career journey in 2001 and uses her leadership experience to inform the teaching around leadership and service improvement. She teaches a range of learners from Foundation Degree level to Master's students on both Nursing and Paramedic programmes at Teesside University. Mel is passionate about facilitating effective leadership and sees this as a key determinant of high quality care for service users.

Caryll Overy is Lecturer/Practitioner for BSc (Hons) Paramedic Practice, University of Brighton, and Learning and Development Lead South East Coast Ambulance NHS Foundation Trust. As an ambulance employee for 20 years, Caryll has experience of how conflict can influence behaviours and morale within the paramedic field. Now working as a university lecturer/practitioner, Caryll has responsibility for delivery of conflict resolution education to student paramedics and in-service staff. Through her role she has explored the widespread connotations of conflict, and appreciates how personal and professional development of individuals in this field could benefit the paramedic profession.

Marion Richardson joined the Ambulance Service in 1986 and qualified as a paramedic in 1992. She has held many posts in the Ambulance Service, including Ambulance Tutor and Divisional Education Lead. Marion left the Ambulance Service in 2009 and is now a Senior Lecturer at Teesside University and is the programme leader for the Foundation Degree in Paramedic Science and the Undergraduate BSc (Hons) Paramedic Programme. The benefits of team-working within the NHS, such as improved patient care, and the opportunity to raise paramedics' professional status within the NHS have fuelled Marion's interest in working as a team and group dynamics.

Paul Street, EdD, MSc, PGDE, BSc (Hons) DipN (Lond), RGN, EN, is a Teaching Fellow in the Faculty of Education and Health, University of Greenwich. He is a qualified nurse and has developed a broad background in clinical practice, practice development and education. He believes that patient care should be truly individualized and based on the best possible evidence. Paul teaches across a range of courses for paramedics and nurses from pre-registration to doctoral levels. This includes subjects such as clinical skills, communication, professional issues, research and teacher preparation. He feels that communication is the cornerstone of practice for all healthcare professionals and thus is of vital importance for patients, colleagues and organizations alike.

Surinder Walia, MSc Leadership & Management in Health, MA HE, PG(Dip) HE, BSc, Cert Man, RGN, EN Myers Briggs trainer (MBTI) 1 & 2, is Deputy Head in the Department of Acute and Continuing Care, School of Health and Social Care, University of Greenwich, and has been a Senior Lecturer since July 2006, prior to which she spent five years as a Lecturer/Practitioner in Medical Nursing. She is responsible for delivering the specialist leadership and management teaching across the pre-registration nursing and paramedic curriculum, in addition to the post-registration specialist courses. Surinder's professional background is in cancer nursing and she has worked in lead positions within acute cancer/haematology/medical settings. Prior to her present position, she held a lecturer practitioner post for five years. Surinder's main interest is in clinical leadership and management within the NHS.

How to use this book

The book has several features that will make it a more useful resource.

The book starts with numerous paramedic clinicians' answers to a standard set of questions relating to leadership. These are presented and termed *paramedic profiles* throughout the text. The reader is able to directly compare the leadership responsibilities and the role of a paramedic to that of a specialist paramedic, for example. It is hoped that this will demonstrate to the reader how the drive to improve the standard of leadership across the NHS is being implemented in the paramedic profession throughout the UK Ambulance Service Trusts.

It must be recognized that the paramedic profiles may vary slightly from Ambulance Trust to Trust, depending on local requirements of personnel operating in these specific roles. In addition, where relevant, the individual chapters make reference to the paramedic profiles and the link is made for the reader between the theory and the reality of role and service delivery. This approach is unique to any leadership book to date and we hope the reader will benefit from the merging of the theory with the reality of leadership in Ambulance Trusts throughout the UK.

A feature entitled *Reflection: points to consider* is included where the author wishes to encourage the reader to reflect on working within the organization or on their experiences or to relate their experience to the theory being discussed.

Self-evaluation exercises are included in many chapters. These encourage the reader to take action to enhance their understanding of the subject being discussed. Many of the exercises refer to Department of Health online resources and many contain a web link to the NHS Leadership Academy's online self-assessment tools.

Case studies are included in all chapters where the author would like the reader to reflect on the theory discussed and think about it in relation to a practice situation.

Acknowledgements

Thanks to the team at OUP, who believed in this text and its editors enough to commission it.

To our colleagues and friends who agreed to add to their already busy workloads to contribute to this text, your commitment, expertise and ability to meet deadlines have been invaluable – thank you.

Our thanks go to Calum Burnett, Stephen Hines, Kath Jennings, John Martin, Professor Andy Newton, James Rouse, Andy Sharman, and Andy Swinburn.

Introduction

Amanda Blaber and Graham Harris

The UK National Health Service (NHS) is most definitely at the centre of controversy at the time of writing. The amount of recommendations made by the Francis Inquiry (Mid Staffordshire NHS Foundation Trust Inquiry, 2013) and the speed with which subsequent recommendations from the government are being published are overwhelming and a significant challenge for NHS Trusts to implement. The scrutiny of all who work in the NHS is unprecedented, with media stories occurring on a least a weekly basis. There is no doubt that until the next election (at least) the NHS will be at the very pinnacle of the political agenda and a major part of political manifestos in the lead-up to the next General Election. It is appropriate then that this book examines some of the key themes within the Francis Inquiry's recommendations and the most recent study, *Patients First and Foremost: The Government's Initial Responses to the Francis Inquiry*, published in March 2013 (DH 2013b).

In summary, the Francis Report (DH 2013a) did the following:

- examined 1 million pages of evidence;
- heard from 250 witnesses;
- had 139 days of oral hearings;
- produced a 1700-page report with 290 recommendations;
- cost £13 million.

Contrary to what the media may have us believe, the Inquiry looked at broader monitoring systems and processes that led or contributed to the failures *and not* at individual patient cases or the internal running of the Trust. It is clear to see why other NHS Trusts are reeling at the Inquiry's recommendations, as processes and systems are likely to be somewhat similar in other NHS Trusts across England and the UK as a whole. From the report's findings, Francis has identified eight themes that require urgent improvement, though recognizing that this will not be achieved in a matter of weeks, but months and years. One of the key themes is: *Leadership*.

The Secretary of State's statement to the House of Commons set out a five-point plan in *Patients First and Foremost: The Government's Initial Response to the Francis Inquiry*:

1. Preventing problems.

2. Detecting problems quickly.

3. Taking action promptly.

4. Ensuring robust accountability.

5. Ensuring staff are trained and motivated.

All of the above points are described in a little detail and work-streams for each point are due to report in 2014. What is significant is the potential role of clinical leadership in each of the five points. NHS managers and team leaders need the candour of frontline staff and *paramedics* in order to achieve each of the points mentioned above. The NHS Leadership framework, released in 2011 has been re-examined, after a relatively short period of time, in order to reflect the recommendations made by the Francis Report. The new Healthcare Leadership Model was released in November 2013 and consists of nine leadership dimensions:

1. Leading with care.

2. Inspiring shared purpose.

3. Evaluating information.

4. Sharing the vision.

5. Connecting our service.

6. Engaging the team.

7. Holding to account.

8. Developing capability.

9. Influencing for results.

For each dimension, leadership behaviours are described on a four-part scale, ranging from 'essential' through 'proficient' and 'strong' to 'exemplary'. More detailed information can be found at www.leadershipacademy. nhs.uk/leadershipmodel. It is clear that leadership will be central to the implementation of the five-point plan and the numerous recommendations made by the Francis Report.

So how might this potentially affect the paramedic profession throughout the UK? All of the Inquiry recommendations were mainly based on hospital systems. These would include the pre-/out-of-hospital care pathways of the paramedic profession. There has been some disquiet that community services were not wholly included in the Inquiry and that this may have set back the improvement of community services for at least 3–5 years with the focus of politicians being on hospital services. However, the recent media attention given to 111 services and the discussion around charging for GP appointments, highlight that attention can switch very quickly. The wider NHS needs to learn from both the Francis Report and *Patients First and*

Foremost and failure to examine their own systems, services and quality may be at their peril. The professional body has included a section on clinical leadership within the third edition of the *Paramedic Curriculum* (COP 2013).

So, to conclude, ambulance services, by nature of their patient contact are the frontline of the NHS and will come under similar scrutiny from internal or external organizations. It is incumbent on all registrants to examine their own practices, in light of the government's five-point plan and take responsibility and lead from inside the organization. This may be the only way that the NHS is able to really put patients *first and foremost* and for this particular aspect of patient care not be just rhetoric but be the *leader*.

Editors' note

Throughout the text, there are many references made to the 2011 Leadership Framework. As mentioned in the above Introduction, readers need to be aware that this framework has been re-structured and published in November 2013 as the 'Healthcare Leadership Model'. The previous Leadership Framework refers to the many 'essentials' of leadership and remains useful for professional development. The Leadership Academy website is where all changes in NHS leadership focus are made public, the editors strongly recommend readers to regularly visit the website to keep abreast of updates.

References

CoP (College of Paramedics) (2014) *Paramedic Curriculum Guidance*, 3rd edn. Bridgwater: The College of Paramedics.

Department of Health (2013a) *Report of the Mid Staffordshire NHS Foundation Trust Public Inquiry: Executive Summary* (The Francis Report). London: TSO.

Department of Health (2013b) *Patients First and Foremost: The Government's Initial Responses to the Francis Inquiry*. London: TSO.

Mid Staffordshire NHS Foundation Trust Public Inquiry (2013) *Report of the Mid Staffordshire NHS Foundation Trust Public Inquiry*. Executive Summary. Chaired by Robert Francis QC. London: TSO.

NHS Leadership Academy (2011) *The Leadership Framework*. Leeds: NHS Leadership Academy.

NHS Leadership Academy (2013) *Healthcare Leadership Model: The Nine Dimensions of Leadership Behaviour*. Leeds: NHS Leadership Academy.

Paramedic profiles

Introduction

Numerous profiles of paramedic clinicians' roles have been collated in this chapter. These profiles demonstrate the wide range of roles, expectations and variety in job descriptions that exist throughout the UK. While not exhaustive, these profiles have been used by the authors of subsequent chapters to illustrate theoretical points, in an attempt to bring the theory to life for the reader and apply it directly to the paramedic sphere of practice. It is clear when reading the profiles that differences in application of the paramedic role exist and this brings with it additional issues when staff move from Trust to Trust. The questions asked within the profiles are standard, so the reader can clearly see the differences in role expectations and application.

In this section we profile a range of paramedic roles:

1. Student paramedic profile

2. Paramedic – clinical role profile

3. Clinical advice paramedic – hear and treat profile

4. Specialist paramedic – paramedic practitioner profile

5. Specialist paramedic – Helicopter Emergency Medical Services profile

6. Advanced paramedic profile

7. Consultant paramedic profile

8. Clinical Director profile

1. Student Paramedic Profile

Q. What is the usual size of your team?

A. *As a student paramedic, the team or crew usually consists of three people.*

Q. Describe the time of day that you work, e.g. times of various shifts? 9–5 p.m.? On call?

A. *Various shift patterns, most commonly, day shifts 6:30–18:30, nights 18:30–06:30 or a link shift 9:00–21:00.*

Q. Description of role, e.g. day-to-day duties.

A. *Observe and support the senior clinician up to but not beyond my skill set as a student paramedic.*

Q. Main responsibilities? Please list them and state if this is different from your job description.

A. *Usually responsible for patient paperwork, undertaking minor, non-invasive clinical duties, for example, baseline observations.*

Q. Provide examples of the types of decisions you make on a daily basis: autonomous, joint, non-applicable, etc.

A. *During my first two years of study I would say this question was non-applicable as decisions were usually made without my input. However, during my third year after staff had gained trust and confidence in me, my ideas were sought more often. Once again, usually on minor issues, such as how best to use manual handling equipment or techniques.*

Q. Explain your leadership and managerial role with your crew/team/other students.

A. *My only experience of leadership over other students has been in scenario situations when nominated by assessors.*

Q. Explain your leadership and managerial responsibilities within the organization, if relevant or appropriate.

A. *Not applicable.*

Q. Would you describe yourself as an autonomous practitioner/leader/manager? Please expand your answer to explain your decision.

A. *Not at this moment in time, as a student, I am working under the guidance of a more senior qualified paramedic.*

Q. Please comment about the value (or not) of the paramedic educator (PEd).

A. *PEds, if fully committed to their students and the responsibilities that accompany the role, are vital to the development and success of the student. I personally have had experience with brilliant PEds and not so brilliant PEds.*

With PEds who have become disillusioned with the role, it places a huge amount of extra unnecessary stress on the student, this is obviously extremely unhelpful. On the other hand, with a good PEd, the transition from first-year student through to third-year student can be made smooth and enjoyable and provides a successful learning environment.

Q. What are the most valuable things about a PEd?

A. *Availability, advanced skill sets, wealth of experience, with regards to both clinical experience and dealing with patients through effective communication.*

Increased knowledge of the paramedic profession, patience, and they provide an outlet for concerns that arise in the clinical arena that may not be relevant in the academic setting.

PEds need to be: welcoming, patient, assertive, understanding and willing.

Q. What resources are available to you during the course of your work?

A. *As student paramedics we have access to university resources, for example, online library and NHS Athens. We can also access the 'staff zone' for all ambulance staff within our area of study. This includes updates, clinical policies, trust policies, etc.*

2. Paramedic Profile

Q. What is the usual size of your team?

A. *I usually work as part of a two-person crew on an ambulance. My crewmate may be a paramedic, a technician or now an emergency care assistant.*

Q. Describe the time of day that you work.

A. *Usually work 12-hour shifts: earlies, lates or nights. Shift rotas vary at different stations. Rotas are calculated to ensure an average of 37.5-hour working week across the number of weeks of the rota.*

Q. Description of role, e.g. day-to-day duties.

A. *Clinical leadership: conduct patient assessment, including interpretation of 12-lead ECG when appropriate. Select and apply in each instance the appropriate patient care procedures in accordance with the current guidance and policies. Liaise with other health professionals and communicate complex information to all levels, both internally and externally. Identify developmental opportunities within the work context and take part in activities which lead to personal and professional development.*

Subject to my level of competency and stage of my career, I would be clinically responsible for monitoring the actions, clinical interventions and treatments carried out by other Trust staff, including student paramedics.

Identify and report to the appropriate authority incidents of risk, neglect, abuse or endangerment to vulnerable adults and children.

Q. Main responsibilities? Please list them and state if this is different from your job description.

A. *If I am the senior clinician on scene, then I have clinical responsibility for the service users' needs. The presence of higher qualified healthcare professionals has a bearing on the degree of responsibility expected.*

Q. Provide examples of the types of decisions you make on a daily basis.

A. *Clinical decisions are rarely made unanimously. There is collaboration between the crew and any other healthcare professional present, as well as with the patient and significant others on scene (or even on the telephone). Clinical decisions may relate to whether or not to transfer a patient to hospital, which treatment centre, if any, is most appropriate. Specialist treatment centres for strokes, arrhythmias, myocardial infarction and major trauma may be selected by the paramedic.*

Q. Explain your leadership and managerial role within your crew/team.

A. *I take a leadership role as attendant or lead clinician paramedic. This is done via playing a mentoring role, leading by example or by gently challenging behaviour not conducive to best practice. I encourage participation and contribution from patients, relatives and from my crewmate to enhance harmony and facilitate the care pathway selected.*

Q. Explain your leadership and managerial responsibilities within the organization, if relevant or appropriate.

A. *From my employer's perspective, I have no managerial or team leader responsibilities, however, as a paramedic, I accept that I have a clinical leadership responsibility for my service users.*

Q. Would you describe yourself as an autonomous practitioner/leader/manager? Please expand your answer to explain your decision.

A. *I would describe myself as an autonomous practitioner. Decisions are made together with my colleague(s), patients and relatives or carers and always in the best interest of the service user.*

Q. What resources are available to you during the course of your work?

A. *Ambulance clinical guidelines. Radio communications with the specialist staff available in the Emergency Operations Centre is also a source of information.*

Q. Does the role you hold bring in any revenue to your employer? If yes, approximately how much per annum?

A. *My employer receives funding for providing the 999 and urgent care service, to which I provide input in my daily duties.*

Q. Do you have the autonomy to influence or dictate the Vision and Strategy of paramedics employed within your organization? If so, how has this been achieved or implemented?

A. *Currently there are many changes and challenges facing paramedic practice. I have no direct input into strategic organizational planning.*

3. Clinical Advice Paramedic – Hear and Treat Profile

Comment: the paramedics engaged by my Trust for this role are Agenda for Change (AFC) pay band 6 managers, however, this does not necessarily imply that they are educated and trained to academic level 6.

Q. What is the usual size of your team?

A. *The team comprises of up to six on duty at any time.*

Q. Describe the time of day that you work.

A. *Full 24-hour rotating shifts, earlies, lates and nights.*

Q. Description of role, e.g. day-to-day duties.

A. *Oversee the clinical leadership of the team in providing support to operational staff.*

Q. Main responsibilities? Please list them and state if this is different from your job description.

A. *Provide leadership and support to operational clinical staff in making clinically sound decisions for patients regarding their clinical treatment, and, where necessary, transport to appropriate destinations, or access to other care pathways.*

Communicate effectively and sensitively with other allied health professionals and Primary Care Trusts, to ensure the most appropriate care pathway is accessed for the patients' needs.

Proactively work with operational paramedics to promote cohesive working and good teamwork.

Gaining consent from callers and encouraging them to follow advised course of action, and recording an accurate and comprehensive log of decisions and actions.

Q. Provide examples of the types of decisions you make on a daily basis.

A. *Is a patient safe to leave home? Can a drug be administered outside of UK Ambulance Clinical Guidelines? Can I treat/transport this patient against his/her will? Where is the most appropriate destination for this patient? What is the most appropriate form of transport? How soon will they need transport?*

Q. Explain your leadership or managerial role within your crew/team.

A. *I am a Band 8 manager, supervising clinical activities of the team. The team works semi-autonomously with priorities (talking to patients, crews) directed by the operational demands.*

Q. Explain your leadership and managerial responsibilities within the organization, if relevant or appropriate.

A. *The team leads in as much as they need to be role models for decision-making. They manage to the extent of reminding/advising operational staff of the correct policy to follow, or allowing them to step outside of that policy.*

Q. Would you describe yourself as an autonomous practitioner/leader/ manager? Please expand your answer to explain your decision.

A. *Yes. Although support is available from other managers and clinicians (up to medical consultant level), the adviser is expected to be able to resolve the majority of questions.*

Q. What resources are available to you during the course of your work?

A. *Significant amount of electronic database access, including NICE guidelines.*

Q. Does the role you hold bring in any revenue to your employer? If yes, approximately how much per annum?

A. *Some commissioned funds, especially in palliative care, use of alternate care pathways. No direct chargeable income.*

Q. Do you have the autonomy to influence or dictate the Vision and Strategy of paramedics employed within your organization? If so, how has this been achieved or implemented?

A. *Yes, particularly around use of appropriate care pathways.*

4. Specialist Paramedic – Paramedic Practitioner Profile

Q. What is the usual size of your team? Do you work alone? As part of a crew/small team or part of a larger team?

A. *There are six paramedic practitioner/specialist paramedics in Primary Care in our team, but we always work alone.*

Q. Describe the time of day that you work.

A. *We work 12-hour shifts (07:15–19:15 or 19:15–07:15) with a 37.5-hour contract on a rota covering 24/7.*

Q. Description of role, e.g. day-to-day duties.

A. *We work on a rapid response vehicle (RRV) and are part of the cover plan and therefore undertake a lot of roadside cover and respond to all categories of call. We therefore carry out all the duties a normal paramedic does on a RRV with the additional responsibility of giving telephone advice to, and taking referrals from, all operational staff (paramedics, technicians and emergency care support workers/ emergency care assistants).*

Q. Main responsibilities? Please list them and state if this is different from your job description.

A. *Briefly, but slightly more in depth. We are expected to carry out and record an in-depth patient examination using the medical model (presenting complaint (PC), history of presenting complaint (HPC), past medical history (PMHx), drug/medication history, including allergies (DMHx), social/family history (SFHx), IMP and PLAN) including full body system assessments (respiratory, cardiac, neurological, abdominal, ENT and musculoskeletal).*

Diagnosis and treatment including pharmacological intervention when appropriate (such as antibiotic therapy) under Patient Group Directives (PGDs).

Wound care (cleaning, suturing, steri-stripping, gluing and dressing).

Direct referral to hospital specialties (on-call medics, surgeons, ENT, maxillo-facial and paediatrics) or GP review.

Demonstrate personal accountability in everyday practice and have an understanding of their responsibility for staff to whom they delegate actions, and be expected to adopt a flexible attitude to take account of the changing needs of the service as dictated by patient and organizational needs.

Q. Provide examples of the types of decisions you make on a daily basis: autonomous, joint, non-applicable, etc.

A. *We are classed as fully autonomous clinicians and are therefore expected to treat and refer or treat and discharge when appropriate. Some brief examples: undertake a cranial nerve assessment following a head injury and make a clinical decision whether the patient is safe to be kept at home or needs to be admitted. Undertake urinalysis to assess if a patient has a UTI, commence antibiotic treatment under PGDs following diagnosis and again, decide if it is clinically safe for the patient to stay at home and arrange for GP follow up.*

Q. Explain your leadership and managerial role within your crew/team.

A. *I have the additional leadership responsibility of giving telephone advice to, and taking referrals from all operational staff (paramedics, technicians and emergency care support workers/emergency care assistants).*

Clinical leader, unless a more senior/specialist professional was on scene.

Q. Explain your leadership and managerial responsibilities within the organization, if relevant or appropriate.

A. *We have no specific leadership or managerial role within the organization but are encouraged to undertake a mentorship role after completing an additional university-based Practice Educator (PEd) credited module.*

Uniquely, however, the only person who has the same, or higher clinical skill level and can therefore provide any clinical leadership is the Clinical Director or Operations/Consultant paramedic within my organization.

Q. Would you describe yourself as an autonomous practitioner/leader/manager? Please expand your answer to explain your decision.

A. *I would describe myself as an autonomous practitioner.*

Q. What resources are available to you during the course of your work?

A. *Currently (but this is in the process of being reviewed due to the cost implications), we are issued with a personal kit, including a PP bag containing an ophthalmoscope, otoscope, blood glucose kit, SpO2 probe, tuning fork, reflex hammer, Littman stethoscope, urinalysis sticks, a selection of wound dressings, and wound care kit. We also have 12-lead ECG capabilities, 30+ Patient Group Directive drugs, in addition to the UK Ambulance Clinical Guidelines drugs, and a mobile phone to make and receive unlimited calls.*

Q. Does the role you hold bring in any revenue to your employer? If yes, approximately how much per annum?

A. *Not as far as I'm aware.*

Q. Do you have the autonomy to influence or dictate the Vision and Strategy of paramedics employed within your organization? If so, how has this been achieved or implemented?

A. *No, not in this role.*

5. Specialist Paramedic – Helicopter Emergency Medical Services Profile

Q. What is the usual size of your team?

A. *The HEMS team consists of four members; two clinical personnel (doctor/paramedic) and two flying personnel (pilot/co-pilot).*

Q. Describe the time of day that you work

A. *The HEMS day shift is 0700–1900 and the night shift 1900–0700. All HEMS members are 24 hours on call to respond to major incidents.*

Q. Description of role, e.g. day-to-day duties.

A. *The HEMS paramedic's role is to work in partnership with a doctor as part of a specialized medical/trauma team bringing critical care skills to the patient at point of illness/injury.*

Working as part of the team within the Emergency Operation Centre (EOC), identifying patients within a pre-defined geographical location, who will benefit from a HEMS team response.

The dispatch, tasking and activation of all HEMS teams by air/land. The deployment of all other physician-based responses.

Providing clinical advice to all pre-hospital care providers and staff within the EOC.

Q. Main responsibilities? Please list them and state if this is different from your job description.

A. *Assist doctors with safe pre-hospital anaesthesia, procedural sedation and thoracotomy procedures. Perform and assist with advanced pleural drainage and blood transfusions, and provide on-scene and remote clinical support to all pre-hospital care providers.*

Ensure all triage decisions of trauma patients are correct at all times and in accordance with the established trauma network.

Liaise and communicate with all emergency services and non-emergency parties on-scene.

Manage other physician-based responses during high demand, mass casualty incidents, and major incidents.

Communicate effectively with other air ambulance providers in providing complete and robust clinical cover when needed.

Provide continued participation in clinical governance, research, presentations and personnel development.

Q. Provide examples of the types of decisions you make on a daily basis: autonomous, joint, non-applicable, etc.

A. *Dispatch and tasking of the HEMS team. Working in EOC the HEMS paramedic has to decide whether to activate the aircraft/car to patients or not. These decisions are based on combinations of information gathered from the caller/crews and experience of the HEMS paramedic.*

Safety decisions are made on the following: to treat patients in their current position or remove to a nearby location; securing and ensuring safety of vehicles, power lines, machinery, equipment and fluid on scene; ensuring the transportation of the patient by aircraft or ambulance is safe.

Patient treatment and triage: making joint decisions with the doctor on the correct clinical plan for each patient encountered. This includes ensuring priority clinical needs are addressed first. Ensuring patients are triaged to the correct hospital depending on their injuries and definitive care requirements.

Q. Explain your leadership and managerial role within your crew/team.

A. *As a HEMS paramedic I need to demonstrate leadership skills in all pre-hospital care activities. The main leadership and managerial skills all come into play when on-scene with a patient. I will commonly need to lead and manage a small or large team, resources and other emergency services while simultaneously being a strong patient advocate.*

Q. Explain your leadership and managerial responsibilities within the organization, if relevant or appropriate.

A. *The HEMS paramedic leadership responsibilities centre on the following: safety issues; patient assessment; team management; equipment application/maintenance/storage; invasive procedures; teaching; communications; EOC dispatch; clinical advice; triage decisions, and project management.*

Q. Would you describe yourself as an autonomous practitioner/leader/manager? Please expand your answer to explain your decision.

A. *As a HEMS paramedic, I am required to act as an autonomous practitioner and leader. This would include emergency operations centre (EOC) dispatch and tasking, patient assessment, treatment and triage decisions, which all centre on autonomous paramedic practice. During mass casualty incidents, the HEMS paramedic will be expected to work independently triaging and treating patients as necessary.*

When on scene the HEMS paramedic needs excellent leadership skills in driving the scene forward and minimizing on-scene times. To enable this to happen, the HEMS paramedic has to organize the team appropriately, matching tasks to correctly skilled persons, while ensuring the team is working together to achieve patient-centred end goals.

Q. What resources are available to you during the course of your work?

A. *Expert clinical advice, assistance and teaching from doctors, surgeons and medical consultants.*

Comprehensive governance and debriefing sessions on safety, treatment plans, patient diagnosis, outcomes and pathophysiology, injury patterns, and triage decisions.

Post-mortem access. Continuous moulage training. Morbidity and mortality discussions. Pre-hospital research support.

6. Advanced Paramedic Profile

Q. What is the usual size of your team?

A. *In my Trust, Advanced paramedics work as part of an organization-wide team comprising of approximately 50 members. Each Advanced paramedic clinically leads and supports a team of Senior paramedics, who in turn lead a wider staff group of 60–80. This larger team will comprise of operational managers, paramedics and emergency medical technicians (EMTs).*

Concerning patient care responsibilities and duties, Advanced paramedics respond as a lone (solo) responder.

Q. Describe the time of day that you work, e.g. times of various shifts. 9–5 p.m.? On-call?

A. *The shift systems comprise of 24-hour shifts varying between 8-, 10- and 12-hour shifts.*

Q. Description of role, e.g. day-to-day duties.

A. *Provide assessment and management of a wide spectrum of patients utilizing relevant evidence-based practice.*

When attending patients, be the senior [paramedic] clinician and undertake this role by having responsibility for the treatment provided to patients and the clinical practice of all paramedics band 6 and below.

Respond to and receive patients with undifferentiated and undiagnosed problems, including responding to 999 and urgent requests for clinical assessment.

Provide face-to-face and remote clinical advice to Senior paramedics in relation to clinical care and alternative care in the community. Provide an advanced clinical assessment of a wide range of minor illness and minor injuries and critically ill patients and be willing to develop skills with the requirements of the service.

Know their limits in relation scope of practice and recognize when a requirement exists to refer patient to, or seek advice from, a Consultant paramedic or any other relevant senior healthcare professional, including a medical professional.

Q. Main responsibilities? Please list them and state if this is different from your job description.

A. *Ensure clinical standards are met and exceeded at all times and ensure Senior paramedics and their respective teams operate within the agreed latest clinical guidelines and any local Trust clinical protocols and procedure.*

Monitoring individual performance of staff within the team of Senior paramedics and provide feedback through a structured peer review process on issues in relation to clinical decisions, treatment and outcomes of clinical performance indicators and mentorship and support their respective teams.

Q. Provide examples of the types of decisions you make on a daily basis: autonomous, joint, non-applicable, etc.

A. *These vary on the operational requirements but include a mixture of autonomous and joint, depending on the incident, and/or patient needs. However, they do include clinical advice for paramedics and operational staff and greater autonomous decision-making.*

Termination of resuscitation attempts in non-conventional circumstances. Treatment locations. Capacity to consent. Pharmocological interventions over and above that of normal practice guidance.

Q. Explain your leadership and managerial role within your crew/team/organization?

A. *As stated, I have the leadership responsibility for the Senior paramedics and the staff within their team in the organization. Concerning patient care responsibilities and duties, I respond as a lone (solo) responder.*

Q. Explain your leadership and managerial responsibilities within the organization, if relevant or appropriate.

A. *Separate to the responsibilities previously mentioned, I am also responsible for investigating and assessing serious disciplinary and capability cases. Monitoring the performance of Senior paramedics and their respective teams in relation to cardiac arrest, especially in relation to downloads from the defibrillator. Monitoring Patient Report Forms completed by Senior paramedics and their respective teams for quality of completion and adherence to guidelines.*

Q. Would you describe yourself as an autonomous practitioner/leader/ manager? Please expand your answer to explain your decision.

A. *Yes. Working within established practice guidelines Advanced paramedics, I have greater freedom (autonomy) to practise than less qualified paramedics and operational staff. I would suggest they have a great deal of autonomy to manage patients' needs, however, they do not have complete freedom to do as they wish.*

To enable the Advanced paramedic to have the freedom they require to operate, they often consult with peers or medical support to discuss specific course(s) of action, this is supplemented by regular peer review.

Q. What resources are available to you during the course of your work?

A. *Besides the operational resources of the vehicle, emergency equipment, IT and communication equipment, access to Consultant paramedic and other senior healthcare professionals, including a medical professional as required.*

Q. Does the role you hold bring in any revenue to your employer? If yes, approximately how much per annum?

A. *Yes, 600K via Commissioning for Quality and Innovation (CQUIN) investment.*

Q. Do you have the autonomy to influence or dictate the Vision and Strategy of paramedics within your organization? If so, how has this been achieved or implemented?

A. *Yes, working with the Professional Development Lead and Consultant paramedics, Advanced paramedics influence the Vision and Strategy as individuals undertaking research into practice, in working groups focusing on specific topical issues, and as part of commissioning arrangements in each area.*

7. Consultant Paramedic Profile

Q. What is the usual size of your team?

A. *The team consists of 1–50 clinicians.*

Q. Describe the time of day that you work.

A. *Normal office hours, 9–5. Clinical Aspect – operational shift basis.*

Q. Description of role, e.g. day-to-day duties.

A. *My education roles are: education and training, teaching, managing and advancing standards of education, working with HEUs (universities), overseeing continuing professional development (CPD) and learning materials.*

My research and development roles are: managing Research & Development Department; research gatekeeper; undertaking research; Commissioning for Quality and Innovation (CQUIN) Trust Lead.

Q. Main responsibilities? Please list them and state if this is different from your job description.

A. *As above.*

Q. Provide examples of the types of decisions you make on a daily basis;

A. *Consultant Paramedic: a variation of autonomous (practitioner), joint decisions (team and trust managerial), in partnership: set scope of practice, and standards of education for clinical practice.*

Q. Explain your leadership and managerial role within your crew/team.

A. *Clinical delivery of paramedics and other Trust practitioners. Clinical consultation and managerial support, and the implementation and introduction of new developments.*

Q. Explain your leadership and managerial responsibilities within the organization, if relevant or appropriate.

A. *Ensure that clinical quality is delivered and achieved, and I also have responsibility for clinical audits.*

Q. Would you describe yourself as an autonomous practitioner/leader/manager? If yes, please expand your answer to explain your decision.

A. *As above. This incorporates and includes use of specialized knowledge to critically analyse, evaluate and synthesize new and complex ideas that are at the most advanced frontier of paramedic practice.*

Q. What resources are available to you during the course of your work?

A. *Individual knowledge, expertise and skills. Knowledge, expertise and skills of team members. Organizational resources including specialist knowledge and skills.*

Q. Does the role you hold bring in any revenue to your employer? If yes, approximately how much per annum?

A. *Yes. £5 million per annum.*

Q. Do you have the autonomy to influence or dictate the Vision and Strategy of paramedics employed within your organization? If so, how has this been achieved or implemented?

A. *Yes, contributing, undertaking and participating in strategic levels of the Trust's Visions and Values, and clinical audit of paramedic practice.*

8. Clinical Director Profile

Q. What is the usual size of your team?

A. *Approximately 2400.*

Q. Describe the time of day that you work

A. *The position is a 24/7, 365-day a year post, technically described as 37.5 hours per week.*

Q. Description of role, e.g. day-to-day duties.

A. *The Clinical Director is primarily responsible for maintaining and improving the clinical effectiveness and operational performance of the service, with reference to acceptable standard(s) as determined by NHS performance measures and other relevant agencies.*

The candidate will be a registered paramedic [HCPC] who has reached consultant paramedic level and will therefore also be responsible for professional leadership, with limited responsibilities in respect of the remaining consultant paramedic domains [expert clinical practice, teaching, research and service development]. It is recognized that these aspects of the role, while important, in terms of retaining currency, given the key nature of this leadership role, cannot be afforded the full commitment of time given the primacy of the Director function.

Q. Main responsibilities? Please list them and state if this is different from your job description.

A. *As described, totally responsible for all key result areas, including the professional leadership and management of all clinical operational staff, to ensure deliver high quality and timely services to patients.*

The delivery of high performance operational services to agreed performance, financial, quality standards, including Emergency Despatch Field Operations and other related functions.

The development and implementation of 'high performance' methodologies to ensure efficient delivery of operational services with demonstrable improvement in productivity and quality measures Intrinsic to these duties is a commitment to quality management improvement techniques, audit and evaluation.

The development and implementation of strategies to provide a wide range of mobile health services that meet the diverse needs of patients.

Strategy development, with particular emphasis upon the needs of paramedics as Allied Health Professionals, and the alignment of the capabilities offered by these staff with a developing concept of operations that keeps pace with the emerging needs of patients and the Trust. Examples include the continued development and support for specialist Paramedic Practitioners and Critical Care Paramedics, together with other emerging specialist paramedic roles.

Effective Emergency Planning and strategic resilience arrangements, including the provision of specialist operations, such as HART and other capabilities.

Financial management, ensuring that budgetary allocations are not breached and that effective financial controls exist at all levels.

Contribute to commissioning process, providing specialist paramedic insights in the relationships between patient demands, the developing clinical concept of operation, patient safety and the link between resourcing and operational effectiveness. Support and contribute to the development of effective clinical governance arrangements.

Q. Provide examples of the types of decisions you make on a daily basis: autonomous, joint, non-applicable, etc.

A. *The post is characterized by extreme diversity, performance management, strategy, communication with internal and external stakeholders and being accountable to the board, which in practice means performance, money, people, risk, mediated in part through board sub-committee.*

Q. Explain your leadership and/or managerial role within your crew/ team.

A. *Lead, accountability for key result areas previously described.*

Q. Explain your leadership and managerial responsibilities within the organization, if relevant or appropriate.

A. *The professional leadership and management of all paramedics and other clinical operational staff to ensure delivery of high quality and timely services to patients.*

Q. Would you describe yourself as an autonomous practitioner/leader/ manager? Please expand your answer to explain your decision.

A. *Yes. I both practise clinically at Consultant Paramedic level, and as previously described professionally manage lead all paramedics within the organization.*

Q. What resources are available to you during the course of your work?

A. *Essentially all the resources of the Directorate, £86 million, 2400 staff, etc., but in reality only the immediate managerial team which support me. Given that most of the money is already spent on generating unit hour and providing an emergency and urgent service.*

Q. Does the role you hold bring in any revenue to your employer?

A. *The revenue comes from the taxpayer via the commissioners.*

Q. Do you have the autonomy to influence or dictate the Vision and Strategy of paramedics employed within your organization? If so, how has this been achieved or implemented?

A. *Yes, having written the strategy.*

PART 1

Introducing leadership

1 Paramedic leadership and the NHS Clinical Leadership Career Framework

Graham Harris

In this chapter

- Introduction
- The paramedic Leadership and Career Framework
- The NHS Leadership and Clinical Leadership Competency Framework
- The Clinical Leadership Competency Framework (CLCF)
- The link between the Clinical Leadership Competency Framework and professional career development for paramedics
- Historical development
- Current development
- Future development
- Conclusion
- Chapter key points
- References and suggested reading
- Useful website

Introduction

The paramedic profession has evolved and developed from an ideology of providing individuals with extended and advanced airway skills, into a profession that provides the individual with a career structure parallel and equal to the other allied health professionals (AHPs) and non-medical professionals within the National Health Service (NHS). The aim of this chapter is to explore the ethos and concepts of leadership within the paramedic profession which includes the paramedic career framework, and the overarching principles indoctrinated in the Leadership Framework.

The framework provides a consistent approach to leadership development for all staff, including paramedics, in healthcare, irrespective of discipline, role, function or seniority and represents the standard for leadership behaviours to which all staff should aspire. The leadership principles have been expanded upon and embraced into the Clinical Leadership and Competency Framework (CLCF) (NHS Leadership Academy 2011b), which identifies that the focus is on the individual as a leader rather than the processes of leadership.

The CLCF has been incorporated into the Paramedic Curriculum Guidance, College of Paramedics (CoP 2014a), which includes the career framework for paramedics and consists of the following levels: *Student Paramedic, Paramedic, Specialist Paramedic, Advanced Paramedic* and *Consultant Paramedic*. This chapter will discuss each of the recognized career routes; *Clinical, Academic, Managerial* and *Research* (Health and Care Professions Council 2012a). It will also consider and provide an historical perspective regarding the development of the paramedic profession, including a discussion about current career development and considerations for the future. The 2013 Healthcare Leadership Model (NHS Leadership Academy 2013) is to help those who work in health to become better leaders. As it is a newly developed model, there will be a period of adjustment and change, whilst staff work with the model and continue to obtain a more in-depth understanding of how it can be used to benefit the individual and organisation's leadership requirements. The major difference with this model is that it is designed to be more dynamic to mirror the changes in healthcare expectation and delivery as time passes. The present version 1.0 is clearly the starting point of this process, the CLCF (NHS Leadership Academy 2011b) is more widely known and used by clinicians and as such, will be the focus of the discussion.

The paramedic Leadership and Career Framework

Career structures

Clinical

Paramedic practice within the UK has developed clinically from what was originally a *first aid qualification*, through to the present-day individual who has expertise in pre- and out-of-hospital practice, and works at the forefront of their field providing expert clinical care, often managing complex cases either autonomously or as part of a multi-professional healthcare team. In the past 40 years, paramedics have been provided with significant opportunities to progress through increased education and development opportunities, including the transition into higher education (Department of Health 2005), and following registration was the inclusion of the protected title 'Paramedic' (Great Britain 2001). This period was the first opportunity to achieve advanced skills, leading to the present-day ability to become a Director of Clinical Services (College of Paramedics 2008) and clearly demonstrates how paramedics and the profession have developed throughout this period. During this evolution the individual paramedic has developed leadership skills, competencies and expertise that are used in clinical practice and throughout their individual career development. Considerable variations of leadership occur across the profession's career structure, as can be seen in the following excerpts from the profiles:

Student paramedic: My only experience of leadership over other students has been in scenario situations when nominated by assessors.

Paramedic: I take a leadership role as attendant or lead clinician [paramedic]. This is achieved via playing a mentoring role, leading by example or by gently challenging behaviour not conducive to best practice. I encourage participation and contribution from patients, relatives and from my crew mate to enhance harmony and facilitate the care pathway selected.

Clinical advice paramedic: Provide leadership and support to operational clinical staff in making clinically sound decisions for patients regarding their clinical treatment, and, where necessary, transport to appropriate destinations, or access to other care pathways.

Specialist paramedic – paramedic practitioner: I have the additional leadership responsibility of giving telephone advice to, and taking referrals from all operational staff (paramedics, technicians and emergency care support workers/emergency care assistants).

Specialist paramedic – Helicopter Emergency Medical Services: As an HEMS paramedic I need to demonstrate leadership skills in all pre-hospital care activities. The main leadership and managerial skills all come into play when on-scene with a patient. I will commonly need to lead and manage a small or large team, resources and other emergency services while simultaneously being a strong patient advocate.

Advanced paramedic: As stated, I have the leadership responsibility for the senior paramedics and the staff within their team in the organization.

Consultant paramedic: Ensure that clinical quality is delivered. Responsibility for clinical audits.

Director of Clinical Operations: The professional leadership and management of all clinical operational staff to ensure deliver high quality and timely services to patients.

As can be seen from the above excerpts, the leadership responsibility of the paramedic increases with career progression. As of September 2013, there were a total of 19,229 paramedics registered with the regulatory body (HCPC 2013a), the data, however, does not quantify the status or level of paramedic. The Centre for Workforce Intelligence Report (CfWI 2012), however, identified the need for the number of Specialist and Advanced Paramedics to be increased to meet the continuing demands on the profession throughout the UK.

Academic

During the previous decade not only have paramedic education and training moved into higher education (Department of Health 2005), but a considerable number of these programmes in paramedic science/practice (HCPC 2012b) have been managed and delivered by academic paramedics. They deliver a myriad of programmes/courses which presently include; level 5 Diploma Higher Education; level 6 pre- and post-registration BSc (Hons) programmes and level 7 MSc postgraduate programmes. While several hold the position of Principal Lecturer and are professional leads, the profession has to date seen the appointment of a paramedic academic professor.

Management

Throughout the period discussed, to enable paramedics to progress within the NHS and their respective Trust, they had to move away from their clinical role and move into operational management, initially as a first-line manager clinical team leader. In the modern NHS opportunities exist which encourage individuals to develop their leadership ability throughout their career to achieve positions such as Director of Clinical Operations (Profile, 2013), and Director of Paramedic Education and Development (Radmore 2013), but also to further develop their leadership expertise and achieve the post of Chief Executive (Harris 2013).

Research

This stream of the paramedic career framework would benefit from similar achievements as the previously discussed career streams. Notwithstanding this, however, paramedics in the UK and internationally have produced and are producing an extensive amount of research evidence, including that which is published in the profession's monthly clinical publication, *Journal of Paramedic Practice* (JPP). Similar to the academic career route, individual paramedics have progressed through this particular stream and hold professorial appointments (JPP 2013).

As discussed, paramedics have expanded and developed their leadership expertise. Each of the career routes provides paramedics with unique opportunities to develop as a leader. These positions are described in the respective streams in Table 1.1.

Separate from the career framework described, opportunities exist for paramedics to further develop in the clinical arena of practice by undertaking a specialist role. These include further education and training to work in one of the following areas of practice: Hazardous Area Response Team (HART), Urban Search and Rescue (USAR), Helicopter Emergency Medical Services (HEMS), Baby/Neonate Emergency Transfer Service (BETS/NETS) (CoP 2014a), and areas such as Emergency Planning Units (EPU). Within the profession military paramedics are also employed in specialist Medical Emergency Response Teams (MERT) (UK Forces Afghanistan 2011).

Table 1.1   Career framework streams

Clinical	Academic	Management	Research
Paramedic	Lecturer Practitioner/Lecturer	Team Leader	Clinical Trial Paramedic
Specialist Paramedic	Senior Lecturer	Middle Manager	Research Fellow
Advanced Paramedic	Principal Lecturer	Senior Manager	Reader
Consultant Paramedic	Professor	Board/Director level Manager	Professor

Reflection: points to consider

- In which career stream do you currently work or practise?
- At what level are you employed?
- How do you see your career developing?
- Does it include development in your current career framework stream?
- Will it require you to develop in another of the career framework streams?

The NHS Leadership and Clinical Leadership Competency Framework

The definition of leadership provided by Northouse can clearly be related to paramedics, 'a process whereby an individual influences a group of individuals to achieve a common goal' (Northouse 2013: 5). On a daily basis, paramedics influence colleagues, patients, carers, allied health professionals, and medical colleagues in providing the most appropriate care for their patient. History informs us that the most common stereotypic idea of leadership is of the individual, powerful, charismatic leader such as Ghengis Khan, Adolf Hitler and Winston Churchill, all of whom had followers in subordinate roles. These people actually were real-life leaders but their styles of leadership are quite limited and rather outdated and from the modern perspective are seen as poor models for leadership development (NHS Leadership Academy 2011a). The leadership framework provides a consistent approach to leadership development in the NHS, irrespective of discipline or role, and was developed by the National Leadership Council after extensive research and consultation with a wide cross-section of staff, including professional bodies, patients and academics. The framework has subsequently been further refined and developed into the CLCF (NHS Leadership Academy 2011a), which builds upon internationally recognized best practice standards of leadership and incorporates the ethos and principles included in the following:

- The Leadership Qualities Framework (LQF) (NHS Institute for Innovation and Improvement 2005).

- The Medical Leadership Competency Framework (MLCF) (NHS Institute for Innovation and Improvement and Academy of Medical Royal Colleges 2010).
- The Clinical Leadership and Competency Framework (CLCF) (NHS Leadership Academy 2011a).

Each of these documents builds upon the evidence from the previous framework and is linked into the next. The leadership framework and the clinical leadership competency framework are interchangeable regarding the initial five core domains for paramedics at all levels:

- Demonstrating personal qualities.
- Working with others.
- Managing services.
- Improving services.
- Setting direction.

The remaining two domains apply to those paramedics who are in (or are aspiring to) the most senior positions of leadership within the profession or organization (see Figure 1.1).

- Creating the vision.
- Delivering the strategy.

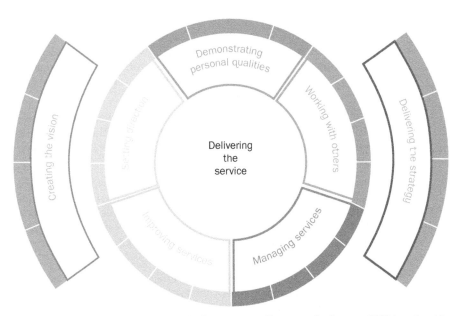

Figure 1.1   The Clinical Leadership Competency Framework. *Source*: NHS Leadership Academy (2011a).

The Clinical Leadership Competency Framework (CLCF)

The CLCF applies to every paramedic at all stages of their professional career journey – from the time they enter formal education and training as a student paramedic, become qualified and registered as a 'paramedic', and throughout their continuing professional development as experienced paramedics, in Specialist, Advanced or Consultant paramedic roles. The CLCF is structured to enable the user to assess how they relate to each of the core domains, and the suggestion is that all healthcare staff, including paramedics, should be competent in the five core domains. The emphasis within the CLCF is on shared responsibility and accountability of all registered professionals (including paramedics) at all levels. The framework is based on the principle of *shared leadership* with the firm understanding that leadership behaviours are not confined to those in senior positions. While there is no entire or familiar pathway to be followed for health professionals, including paramedics, to demonstrate competence and capacity in the domains and subsequent elements, how the individual paramedic does so will vary depending on either their level of expertise and training or the career trajectory of the person. Conversely, all competences should be achieved and verified at each level of career stage. The domains and elements are described below:

- *Demonstrating personal qualities*: Paramedics showing effective leadership need to draw upon their values, strengths and abilities to deliver high standards of care. This requires them to demonstrate ability in: developing self-awareness, managing themselves, continuing personal development (CPD), and acting with integrity.

- *Working with others*: Paramedics show leadership by working with others in teams and networks to deliver and improve services. This requires them to demonstrate ability in: developing networks, building and maintaining relationships, encouraging contribution, and working within teams.

- *Managing services*: Paramedics showing effective leadership are focused on the success of the organization in which they work. This requires them to demonstrate ability in: planning, managing resources, managing people, and managing performance.

- *Improving services*: Paramedics showing effective leadership make a real difference to people's health by delivering high quality services and by developing improvements to services. This requires them to demonstrate ability in: ensuring patient safety, critically evaluating, encouraging improvement and innovation, facilitating transformation, and improving services.

- *Setting direction*: Paramedics showing effective leadership contribute to the strategy and aspirations of the organization and act in a manner consistent with its values. This requires them to demonstrate ability in: identifying the contexts for change, applying knowledge and evidence, making decisions, and evaluating impact.

The remaining two domains apply to those paramedics who are in (or are aspiring to) the most senior positions of leadership within the profession or organization.

- *Creating the vision*: Paramedics in senior positional leadership roles create a compelling vision for the future, and communicate this within and across organizations. This requires them to demonstrate success in: developing the vision for the organization, influencing the vision of the wider healthcare system, communicating the vision, and embodying the vision.

- *Delivering the strategy*: Paramedics in senior positional leadership roles deliver the strategic vision by developing and agreeing strategic plans and ensuring that these are translated into achievable operational plans. This requires them to demonstrate success in: framing the strategy, implementing the strategy, and embedding the strategy.

The HCPC published a position statement on the CLCF (HCPC 2012c) and stated that it is important in helping clinicians to gain a shared understanding of what leadership is. The emphasis on a *shared approach* of all staff members is consistent with the HCPC Standards which emphasize both personal responsibility and the importance of working effectively with others. The HCPC also advises that the CLCF aims to entrench leadership capability and the skills associated with it across the clinical workforce, rather than focusing on a smaller number of clinicians with managerial responsibilities (HCPC 2012c: 3).

The HCPC recommends that many of the skills, attitudes and behaviours described in the CLCF should be well embedded in the Standards of Proficiency (HCPC 2012d) and are well reflected in their Standards of Conduct, Performance and Ethics (HCPC 2012e). However, the HCPC recognizes, within the position statement, that it is important for registrants at the point of entry to have an understanding of the concept of leadership to develop their skills in practice. As a result, a new standard of proficiency has been included in generic Standard 13 which reads: 'understand the concept of leadership and its application to practice' (HCPC 2013a). This change recognizes the importance of every paramedic contributing to the leadership agenda, whether commencing an approved and endorsed programme of education as a student paramedic, or as a registered qualified and experienced paramedic, as there is a requirement to continue to meet the standards to maintain professional registration. In addition, education providers are required to deliver programmes and courses which meet the HCPC Standards of Education and Training (SETs), and Standards of Proficiency (HCPC 2012d, 2013c), and consequently *leadership* must be embedded within the taught curriculum. The guidance document provides examples of how the various levels of practitioners can achieve the domains, and how the CLCF can be incorporated into higher education programmes (NHS Leadership Academy 2011b). The Leadership Academy in the 2013 publication, *NHS Healthcare Leadership Model*, asks for examples of how version 1.0 of the Model has been used in clinical practice, as they would like to collect examples of best practice, highlighting a new chapter in leadership models for the NHS. Many of the domains detailed in the CLCF remain in the 2013 Model, see www.nhsleadershipacademy for more details.

The link between the Clinical Leadership Competency Framework and professional career development for paramedics

Whether as a student paramedic undertaking a programme of pre-registration education, or as a Director of Clinical Operations responsible for 'the professional leadership and management of all clinical operational staff to ensure deliver high quality and timely services to patient', or any of the interim levels of paramedic, every level should understand that there is an inextricable link between leadership and the development of the individual's professional career. To enable the individual paramedic to develop throughout their professional career, they must implement and develop effective leadership by demonstrating competence in all domains and elements of the NHS Leadership Academy (NHS Leadership Academy 2011a). The levels of practitioner identified within the CLCF are related to the relevant level of paramedic as follows:

- Student – pre-registration entry level formal education
  Student Paramedic

- Practitioner – qualified or registered professional
  Paramedic

- Experienced practitioner – practitioner with greater complexity and responsibility in their role.
  Specialist, Advanced, or Consultant paramedic.

As described earlier in the chapter, paramedics at each level are expected to incorporate the respective domains and elements of the clinical leadership competency framework into their practice (NHS Leadership Academy 2011a). The document provides examples of each domain and subsequent elements from both the learning and development opportunity and practice perspectives. A modified description and an example of the learning and development opportunity are provided in Table 1.2. This demonstrates the wide range of opportunity to learn from each individual clinical encounter with colleagues, patients and families.

Domain 1: Demonstrating Personal Qualities

Clinicians/paramedics showing effective leadership need to draw upon their values, strengths and abilities to deliver high standards of care.

Table 1.2   Examples of learning and development opportunities

Student paramedic	Paramedic	Specialist paramedic
Using information from tutors, peers, staff and patients to develop further learning	Obtaining feedback from a range of others in preparation for appraisal	Initiating own 360° feedback to enhance reflective practice
Reflecting on performance in end of term discussion and identifying own strengths and weaknesses	Taking part in peer learning and exploring team and leadership styles and preferences	Using information from psychometric and behavioural measures
Making assessed presentation as part of course and obtaining structured feedback	Taking part in case conferences as part of multidisciplinary and multi-agency team, and obtaining feedback on effectiveness of own contribution	Reflecting on performance in end of term discussion and identifying own strengths and weaknesses
Chairing small group activities and seeking feedback on effectiveness		

Source: NHS Leadership Academy (2011b:12).

Element 1.1 Developing Self-Awareness

1. Recognize and articulate their own values and principles, under-standing how these may differ from those of other individuals and groups.

2. Identify their own strengths and limitations, the impact of their behaviour on others, and the effect of stress on their own behaviour.

3. Identify their own emotions and prejudices and understand how these can affect their judgement and behaviour.

4. Obtain, analyse and act on feedback from a variety of sources.

Case study 1.1

A first-year student paramedic accompanies their practice educator (PEd) to a patient who is seriously ill in their own home, with family present. The family are very anxious, pleading with the paramedic to 'do something' and it is clear the patient is very ill.

The paramedic is thoroughly assessing and treating the patient when the patient goes into cardiac arrest. The student is shocked and does not know what to do, the paramedic crew instigate full and appropriate care. After a significant period of time, the crew call a halt to the resuscitation and pronounce the patient dead. This distressed the student, as they did not have the knowledge or experience to understand the decision-making process and the crew did not have time to explain it, until after the event.

The crew's attention turned to care of significant others and family members, who were obviously distraught and upset.

Despite being proficient at simulated basic life support, the student paramedic felt totally out of their depth, as this was their first experience of real-life resuscitation. The student required a significant amount of debriefing time and reflection, both with the crew and on their own.

The student paramedic throughout their programme or course of pre-registration education will be given opportunities and advice on achieving each of the domains. A potential interpretation of how they might demonstrate effectiveness of Element 1.1 – Developing self-awareness is as follows.

1. *Recognize and articulate their own values and principles, understanding how these may differ from those of other individuals and groups.* On entry to the programme they will bring their own values and principles, which they discover may not be the same as their peers. During practical placements this is confirmed when dealing with patients from various cultures and age spectrum.

2. *Identify their own strengths and limitations, the impact of their behaviour on others, and the effect of stress on their own behaviour.* As highlighted in case study 1.1, in the first year of study, the student had developed the appropriate level of skill in basic life support (BLS) resuscitation, but when confronted with their first cardiac arrest, realized that it is not only the skills, knowledge and scope of practice that are required in advanced life support (ALS), and became stressed when the paramedic mentor terminated the resuscitation procedure and had to console distressed significant others.

3. *Identify their own emotions and prejudices and understand how these can affect their judgement and behaviour.* In case study 1.1, the paramedic mentor suggested to the student that they reflect on the experience. On completing a reflection of the incident, they identified and described their emotions and ascertained the need for particular clinical decisions to be made, which demonstrated their need to modify their behaviour to enable them also to make effective clinical judgements.

4. *Obtain, analyse and act on feedback from a variety of sources.* As they progress through their course of education, the student receives

feedback from peers during role-play, from tutors during simulation, and when undertaking reflection and work-based practice placements. They then act upon the feedback which they analyse to become a competent paramedic.

However, a Consultant paramedic potentially may demonstrate effectiveness for the same element by doing the following.

1. *Recognize and articulate their own values and principles, understanding how these may differ from those of other individuals and groups.* After being appointed to the position of Consultant paramedic in a different NHS Trust, they recognize that their values and principles are not necessarily the same as the paramedics employed by the Trust or as the service users in their new employer's geographical area.

2. *Identify their own strengths and limitations, the impact of their behaviour on others, and the effect of stress on their own behaviour.* They have an MSc in their area of expertise and are currently completing their PhD thesis, however, while this is their clinical strength, they also realize that the majority of their current workforce have not had a similar opportunity to develop, becoming stressed about a new clinical assessment procedure they have implemented into practice.

3. *Identify their own emotions and prejudices and understand how these can affect their judgement and behaviour.* As the Clinical Lead for the Trust complaints procedure, they relate to a paramedic undertaking preceptorship who has been referred, following a complaint for referring a patient to the regional trauma centre. When they were newly registered, there were no such specialist units and this is their area of specialism and they do not want this to affect their judgement.

4. *Obtain, analyse and act on feedback from a variety of sources.* As part of their role they are responsible for reviewing the clinical performance indicators (CPIs) data, and delivering these to the Trust board and external contractual bodies. The feedback from these and other sources have to be analysed and implemented in future practice.

Reflection: points to consider

In relation to Element 1.1 – Developing Self-Awareness and the subsequent four sub-elements:
- What examples would you provide in your current position to demonstrate effectiveness?

Box 1.1   Learning and development activities

Reading and research

Tutor discussion

Mentoring/peer assistance

Simulation

Direct knowledge and skills teaching

Group problem-solving

Scenarios

Patient discussion/patient story

Role-play

Written reflection

Small group activity

Shadowing

Project work

Audit and evaluation

Work based learning.

Source: NHS Leadership Academy (2011b: 38–44).

The guidance document produced by the NHS Leadership Academy (2011b) demonstrates how in the context of clinical leadership the competent paramedic acquires the knowledge, skills, attitudes and behaviours in order to meet each specific competency. It also provides examples of learning and development activities that can be incorporated into existing curriculum activity for student paramedics. These range from individual activities (reflective writing, portfolio development) to those which are undertaken in a collective environment (formal teaching sessions and small group activities) (see Box 1.1).

Reflection: points to consider

- Review the list in Box 1.1 and make a list of the learning and development activities you currently use in your practice.
- Then ask yourself, could you use the remainder in integrating the Clinical Leadership Competency Framework into your existing curriculum or practice?

Historical development

The modern-day paramedic has seen key changes to their practice and profession since the formation of the UK National Health Service (NHS) in 1947. Professional career development has evolved from the early days of a simple first aid qualification and the status of manual workers, through the progression of paramedic education and training which has seen far-reaching improvements in the standards and quality of patient care. Present-day paramedics are established Allied Health Professionals (AHPs) in their own right (Department of Health 2003), with all the responsibilities that such status brings. The following section will consider the historical development of the profession through the early decades, providing a synopsis of the key achievements.

1960s: National vocational qualification

The most important aspect of this decade was the publication of the Millar Report in 1966. The report was in essence two reports, one of which focused on ambulance service equipment, and the other on ambulance training. Prior to the reports, training had been the responsibility of the respective ambulance service. A broader input into the training curriculum was incorporated from other professions, which included medical, nursing and midwifery and mental health. While the reports provided a national standard for equipment and training, the period of preparation was short and dominated by a training focus rather than an educational ethos, and the career development within the ambulance service focused primarily on a vocational route, delivering patient care at basic life support intensity.

1970s: Extended training schemes

This decade commenced with the introduction of the first 'Paramedic' cardiac scheme in Brighton (CoP 2014a), and this was shortly followed by another in Bristol and then others throughout the UK in the early 1970s. These schemes all had small numbers of cohorts and reflected in the main the requirements of local medical opinion. The NHS Reorganisation Act which was totally implemented on the 1st April 1974, transferred all ambulance services, including those with extended paramedic systems, from the control of local authorities to the NHS. As the 'Paramedic' schemes developed during the latter part of the decade, the transition caused a considerable amount of discussion surrounding the advantages of ambulance staff undertaking an extended role.

The Medical Commission on Accident Prevention (MCAP) set up a committee to ascertain the potential of such a role, and the findings were that, as ambulance staff were often first on the scene, it would be logical to train them in advanced resuscitation techniques.

1980s: National paramedic qualification

In the early 1980s, the Department of Health commissioned an analysis into the benefits of implementing these advanced training programmes on a national basis. This resulted in the establishment of a nationwide pilot scheme in 1985 under the national leadership of Roland Furber (College of Paramedics 2014a). The introduction of portable defibrillators also had an influence on the curriculum design with standardized training programmes being delivered in regional training centres, and this included a formal period of in-hospital training. On successful completion of the training programme, the individual received their award from the National Health Service Training Authority (NHSTA), which by the end of the decade had been replaced by the National Health Service Training Directorate (NHSTD).

1990s: Awarding body, higher education and registration

During the early part of the 1990s, the awarding body for ambulance services and the paramedic qualification was transferred to the Institute of Healthcare and Development (IHCD). By the mid-1990s, the weight of the extra paramedic skills caused a number of educationalists to question the worth of the underpinning knowledge base, to enable the paramedic to deliver appropriate patient care into the next century. In 1996, two higher education institutions (HEIs), Hertfordshire and Coventry, formed partnerships with the London and Warwickshire Ambulance Service respectively and developed degree programmes in Paramedic Science, commencing the move for the profession into higher education. The latter part of the decade saw paramedics applying to become registered with the Council of Professions Supplementary to Medicine (CPSM) as the then 12th group of Allied Health Professions (Saunders 1998).

2000s: Professional, Statutory and Regulatory Bodies (PSRBs)

The British Paramedic Association (BPA) was established as the professional body for paramedics in 2000, and following feedback from the membership the title was formally changed to the College of Paramedics (CoP) in 2008. In 2003, the then Health Professions Council (HCPC) was set up as the regulatory body for all allied health professions. A year later the Quality Assurance Agency published the paramedic benchmarking document (QAA 2004). In the same year, the NHS Modernisation Agency launched the introduction of the Emergency Care Practitioner (ECP), which was to pave the way for a new breed of paramedic (NHS Modernisation Agency 2004). In 2005, recommendations were made to merge the ambulance services throughout the UK, which occurred in 2006, and also to move paramedic education and training to higher education-delivered models (Department of Health 2005). The professional body published the first curriculum in 2006 (British Paramedic Association 2006) and the second edition in 2008 (CoP 2008). During the past four decades paramedics have developed from what was an experimental idea into one of the current 16 Allied Health Professions delivering emergency and urgent healthcare to meet the needs of patients in the twenty-first century.

Current development

NHS Ambulance Trusts are implementing preceptorship programmes to enable newly registered paramedics to be inducted into their respective NHS organization (Department of Health 2010a). Work is in progress to enable student paramedics to utilize drugs under the direct supervision of the registered practice educator, except for the controlled paramedic exemptions drugs as described by the Medicines Health Regulatory Authority (MHRA) (MHRA 2013). The *Paramedic Evidence-Based Education Project* report, funded by the College of Paramedics (Lovegrove 2013), and released by Health Education England (HEE), made several recommendations that will have significant impact on the future leadership and development of the profession. In 2012, the HPC became the Health and Care Professions Council (HCPC) and is currently reviewing the Standards of Proficiency for each of the professions (HCPC 2012c), last updated in 2007. The third edition is due for release in June 2014. The professional body has implemented an endorsement scheme for programmes and short courses and has also set up regional groups that deliver continuing professional development events and workshops available to members and non-members. These are delivered by expert paramedics who have developed along the career framework pathway introduced in the professional body's paramedic Career and Competence Framework (CoP 2014b).

Link to Chapter 10 for more on preceptorship.

Future development

At the time of writing, the professional body is undertaking further work regarding paramedics becoming independent prescribers (Department of Health 2010b). This career development will require the individual to undertake a period of further education and development that meets the standards set by the HCPC (2013d). Eligibility to entry to the register for the profession is set to become an all-undergraduate level (College of Paramedics 2014a). This will also bring about the need to ensure that paramedics who do not have a higher education qualification are provided with the prospect of development by undertaking an appropriate programme of higher education as part of their continuing professional development. Further to the earlier discussions in this chapter, there is a need to increase the numbers of Specialist and Advanced paramedics (CfWI 2012). The outcome of the professional body's application to become eligible for the NHS Bursary Scheme (Department of Health 2012) will have a major impact on the development of the profession and potential future members.

Reflection: points to consider

- Consider the career opportunities that have occurred since the professional body was developed in 2000, only 14 years ago.
- Where do you want your career to be in relation to these in 2026?

Conclusion

As discussed, the career framework for paramedics has developed beyond all recognition during the past 40 years, from the initial first aid qualification into the only country in the world that currently requires the individual to be registered to use the title of Paramedic. Those who decide on a career as a paramedic have to undertake a programme of higher education that is approved by the regulatory body (HCPC 2009). The present career structure enables the individual to progress from the initial level, through all the following clinical levels: student paramedic, paramedic, Specialist paramedic, Advanced paramedic, and Consultant paramedic. Separate to these clinical levels are further prospects of developing in specialist units such as: Hazardous Area Response Team (HART), Urban Search and Rescue (USAR), Helicopter Emergency Medical Services (HEMS), Baby/Neonate Emergency Transfer Service (BETS/NETS), or Emergency Planning Units (EPU). If paramedics so choose, they have the option of developing into academia, management or research, with each stream following an individual career framework structure. The decision is yours.

Chapter key points

- The paramedic profession has a specific career framework unique within NHS Trusts.
- There is a clear link between the Clinical Leadership and Competence Framework and paramedics' career development.
- Paramedics need to be familiar with both frameworks and structure their continuing professional development around the domains.
- Varying levels of leadership should be an integral part of any registrant's everyday responsibilities.
- The historical aspect of the role of a paramedic has developed from a vocational training aspect into the present-day higher education curriculum.
- The potential for future career development will be in response to the demands of society, and the ability of the profession to deliver the appropriate care to the patient, in the right place, and at the right time.

References and suggested reading

BPA (British Paramedic Association) (2006) *A Curriculum Framework for Ambulance Education.* Derby: British Paramedic Association/College of Paramedics.

CfWI (Centre for Workforce Intelligence) (2012) *Workforce Risks and Opportunities Paramedics: Education Commissioning Risks Summary from 2012.* Woking: Mouchel Management Consulting Ltd.

CoP (College of Paramedics) (2008) *Paramedic Curriculum Guidance & Competence Framework,* 2nd edn. Derby: College of Paramedics.

CoP (College of Paramedics) (2014a) *Paramedic Curriculum Guidance,* 3rd edn. Bridgwater: The College of Paramedics.

CoP (College of Paramedics) (2014b) Paramedic Career & Competency Framework. Bridgwater. Unpublished (due November 2013).

Department of Health (2003) *The Chief Health Professions Officer's Ten Key Roles for Allied Health Professionals.* London: Department of Health.

Department of Health (2005) *Taking Healthcare to the Patient: Transforming NHS Ambulance Services.* London: Department of Health.

Department of Health (2010a) *Preceptorship Framework for Newly Registered Nurses, Midwives and Allied Health Professionals.* London: Department of Health.

Department of Health (2010b) *Proposals to Introduce Prescribing Responsibilities for Paramedics: Stakeholder Engagement.* London: Department of Health.

Department of Health (2012) *Professional Eligibility for the NHS Bursary Scheme: Call for Evidence.* Leeds: Department of Health.

Great Britain (2001) *Health Care and Associated Professions – Health Professions – The Health Professions Order 2001.* Statutory Instrument 2002 No. 254. London: The Stationery Office.

Harris, L. (2013) Chief Executive and registered paramedic joins the College of Paramedics, *College of Paramedics Newsletter,* 4(2): 12–13.

HCPC (Health and Care Professions Council) (2009) *Approval Process: Supplementary Information for Education Providers.* London: HCPC.

HCPC (Health and Care Professions Council) (2012a) *Continuing Professional Development and Your Registration.* London: HCPC.

HCPC (Health and Care Professions Council) (2012b) Register of approved programmes. Available at: http://www.hpcuk.org/education/programmes/register/index.asp?EducationProviderID=all&StudyLevel=all&ModeOfStudyID=all&professionID=10&Submit.x=38&Submit.y=15 (accessed 20 August 2013).

HCPC (Health and Care Professions Council) (2012c) *Position Statement on the NHS Clinical Leadership Competency Framework (CLCF).* London: HCPC.

HCPC (Health and Care Professions Council) (2012d) *Standards of Proficiency: Paramedics.* London: HCPC.

HCPC (Health and Care Professions Council) (2012e) *Standards of Conduct Performance and Ethics.* London: HCPC.

HCPC (Health and Care Professions Council) (2013a) Number of paramedic registrants. Available at: http://www.hpc-uk.org/aboutregistration/theregister/stats/ (accessed 30 September 2013).

HCPC (Health and Care Professions Council) (2013b) Draft Standards of Proficiency for Paramedics. Unpublished. London: HCPC.

HCPC (Health and Care Professions Council) (2013c) *Standards of Education and Training.* London: HCPC.

HCPC (Health and Care Professions Council) (2013d) *Standards for Prescribing.* London: HCPC.

Journal of Paramedic Practice (2013) The clinical monthly for emergency care professionals. Available at: http://www.paramedicpractice.com/cgi-bin/go.pl/library/issues.html?journal_uid=41 (accessed 25 August 2013).

Lovegrove, M. (2013) *Paramedic Evidence-Based Education Project.* Buckingham: Allied Health Solutions.

MHRA (Medicines Health Regulatory Authority) (2013) *Paramedic Exemptions.* Available at: http://www.mhra.gov.uk/Howweregulate/Medicines/Availabilityprescribingsellingandsupplyingofmedicines/ExemptionsfromMedicinesActrestrictions/Paramedics/index.htm#12 (accessed 4 August 2013).

NHS Leadership Academy (2011a) *Clinical Leadership Competency Framework.* Coventry: NHS Institute for Innovation and Improvement.

NHS Leadership Academy (2011b) *Guidance for Integrating the Clinical Leadership Competency Framework into Education and Training.* Coventry: NHS Institute for Innovation and Improvement.

NHS Leadership Academy (2013) *Healthcare Leadership Model: The Nine Dimensions of Leadership Behaviour.* Version 1.0. Leeds: NHS Leadership Academy. Available at: www.leadershipacademy.nhs.uk/leadershipmodel (accessed 26 November 2013).

NHS Modernisation Agency (2004) *The ECP Report: Right Skill: Right Place; Right Time.* London: COI Communications for the Department of Health.

Northouse, P. G. (2013) *Leadership Theory and Practice,* 6th edn. London: Sage.

QAA (Quality Assurance Agency) (2004) *Paramedic Science: Health Care Programmes. Phase 2.* Gloucester: The Quality Assurance Agency for Higher Education.

Quinn, R. (2004) *Building the Bridge as You Walk on It: A Guide for Leading Change.* San Francisco: Jossey-Bass.

Radmore, A. (2013) *Appointment of Director of Paramedic Education & Development.* London: London Ambulance Service NHS Trust.

Saunders, R. (1998) Yes to state registration: how paramedics are moving towards registered professionals, *Ambulance UK*, 13(4): 206–9.

UK Forces Afghanistan (2011) Medical Emergency Response Team (MERT): 24 hours in pictures. Available at: https://www.google.co.uk/?gws_rd=cr#fp=2332ad6da73a67be&q=Military+MERT+Teams (accessed 25 August 2013).

Useful website

www.collegeofparamedics.co.uk.

2 Paramedic leadership
What is it and who does it?

Paul Jones

Introduction

This chapter focuses on general leadership characteristics and provides an overview of various leadership styles. This should enable you to identify which personal characteristics lead to which style. It looks at some new leadership theories which have recently been advocated for use by the National Health Service (NHS) strategy and it also makes links to paramedic practice and the numerous ambulance service structures which are in existence in the United Kingdom (UK).

It is not the intention of this chapter to offer lists and examples of good and bad leaders throughout history. The many websites and historical recollection texts that are already in existence are available to the reader. This chapter will focus on *who* a leader needs to be if they are to succeed. Not *who* in name but *who* in broader, more holistic terms. It is hoped that by doing this it will challenge you, the reader, to consider who *you* are and to examine whether or not you have the appropriate personality traits and characteristics. As for the *what* element, the chapter intends to focus on what can be achieved in order to develop some of those key, important characteristics that are needed to become a better leader. We will be looking at what being a leader is and how good leadership can be achieved to a higher standard using strategy that exists or alternatively a new strategy that needs to be created.

Modern paramedic leadership styles have developed for a number of reasons in recent years. Many characteristics which used to be perceived as strong, positive traits are now being challenged as dated and no longer aligned with the *politically correct* and *personality savvy* leader who is needed in the professional world of emergency paramedicine. The leadership theories which support these changes have not changed though, so it is worth questioning who it is that has started to interpret these theories in a different way.

The NHS Leadership Strategy was created in order to deliver leadership in a more scientific manner in the UK. By developing plans and agreeing to place patient care at the heart of all healthcare services, leaders are able to ensure realistic translation of these plans as workable SMART plans: Specific, Measurable, Achievable, Realistic, Timely, see Figure 2.1.

The implications of a leadership strategy for those tasked with leading paramedics are now starting to be recognized. This chapter looks at these implications with an open mind, in the hope that this will lead to further broad investigation of the overall strategy. Nonetheless, there will be a specific focus on the paramedic's role.

True links exist between theory and practice. The links can be seen regionally when leaders use narrative story telling (a technique that enables succinct presentation to an audience and connection to those who are

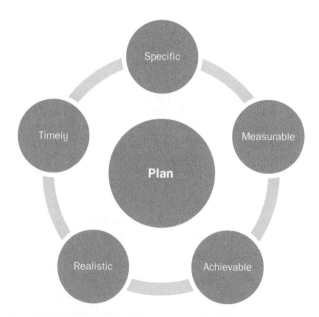

Figure 2.1   The SMART Leadership plan.

like-minded) or social movements to influence their teams. Social movements are groups of people who share values or interests and come together voluntarily to right wrongs (NHS Change Model 2013). Those who lead in this way are engaging and team-focused – more likely to focus on clinical support than on clinical supervision. Yes, granted, there are some paramedics who lead from a perceived position of power, those who theorize about what may or may not be best for those who operationalize and implement their guidance, protocols or policies. Theorizing need not be completely criticized or ruled out as unhelpful. Theory and practice can, and should, be linked intrinsically. A good leader will do this by means of either tacit, unseen skill or alternatively as a deliberate act. Either way, they will do it! If they fail to do so, then as a consequence the risks will become very apparent very quickly. A workforce of paramedics who feel as though their leader is taking the wrong route, will quickly become disillusioned. When this happens, they may stop following the leader, and then who will be the leader when there is no-one left to lead?

Case study 2.1

A road paramedic crew (with supernumerary third-year paramedic student) and solo responder (also a paramedic) requested assistance from the Helicopter Emergency Medical Services (HEMS). After their in-depth assessment, they deemed that their patient required rapid transport to a trauma centre and potential surgical interventions that the paramedics were not able to provide within their skill set. The three paramedics and student had been with the patient for approximately 50 minutes and had instigated treatment, but the patient remained critically ill.

The helicopter, with doctor and Specialist paramedic practitioner on board, landed at the site. After allowing the paramedic who had taken the lead to explain the scene, assessment and treatment, the doctor and the Specialist paramedic practitioner completed their own assessment. During this assessment the patient went into cardiac arrest. The paramedics commenced cardio-pulmonary resuscitation (CPR).

The doctor and the Specialist paramedic practitioner withdrew from the rest of the team, had a whispered discussion and then abruptly returned to the rest of the team and told them to stop CPR.

The paramedic team initially refused to stop CPR. The lead paramedic asked for the rationale to stop CPR (as this conversation had occurred away from the rest of the paramedic team and did not involve them at all) and expressed his disgust and amazement that fellow professionals did not have the courtesy to involve the paramedics in this decision-making for a patient whom they had tried to save for an hour.

The helicopter crew left the scene and left the paramedics and the student angry, frustrated and disillusioned about the leadership of the more senior clinical team.

Case study 2.1 highlights poor clinical leadership, not necessarily in terms of the clinical decision made for the patient, but in the way the paramedics were treated at the scene of this incident. On discussion, the paramedics felt there was a definite position of power over them being taken by the doctor and the Specialist paramedic practitioner. The behaviour of the helicopter team demonstrates this power; whispering, moving aside (away from the paramedics), not involving the paramedics in making the decision, and certainly not valuing their role to this point or their clinical opinions. This example demonstrates the *directing* leadership style discussed in the next section of this chapter. It was not the decision made that was an issue, it was the manner in which the decision was made and the lack of communication between what ended up being two teams. In the patient's best interests, there should have been one united team with excellent communication, explanation of their respective thought processes and joint discussion about the potential decisions to be made.

How different this situation could have been, with supportive coaching and delegating styles of leadership being used within an overarching directive approach, where each professional understood and respected the views of the individuals within the team, despite their varied roles. This would have been a much more positive experience for all concerned and one that would have been a positive learning experience for the student paramedic.

Leadership styles and characteristics

Paramedic leadership can take the form of a number of specific styles developed and noted by many who focus more broadly on NHS leadership. The fundamental concept of dynamic pre-hospital leadership is that no one style of leadership is best in all circumstances. The most successful paramedic leaders are the ones who are able to adapt their style to any given situation, changing as the scene evolves. This consists of four general styles which each have their own distinct characteristics:

- supportive
- coaching
- delegating
- directing.

Supportive

In this style, the leader takes the role of the motivator, leading from the front (Donald Walters 2000). The predominant function of the style is to instil and develop confidence in others. This confidence enables professional independence, autonomy and empowerment. The supportive style is commonly referred to as a *promotional* style as it enables leaders to use persuasion with their staff – encouraging them to have high standards. It also encourages the belief that professional role development is important and should be undertaken continuously. Typically, this style of leadership involves a certain amount of delegation while simultaneously providing the required support. If the support is not offered, then it can create problems of overburden for those being led.

Coaching

This type of leadership style involves a large proportion of contact time and involvement on the part of the leader with the paramedics in the field. Kaye (2005, cited in Goldsmith and Lyons 2006) sees coaching as an executive form of leadership. It is of most benefit to those being led when there are gaps in knowledge, skills or professionalism. This is achieved through demonstration and one-to-one encouragement. For this particular style to be as effective as the leader would want it to be, the paramedic being led needs, first, to *accept* that a gap exists and furthermore to show that they are motivated or driven enough to want to actually fill it!

Delegating

This style places a higher level of responsibility on the shoulders of the paramedic. It has been welcomed by some and criticized by others as it can create the risk of professional burn-out (Health Knowledge Online 2013). From a clinical leader's perspective, they need to recognize their role as the delegator. A strong leader offers guidance and direction but only as and when required by the paramedics themselves.

It also allows the leader to perform in more of a consultancy role than a direct *hands-on* leadership role. It is most effective where there are experienced paramedics who have the ability to function with a high proportion of independence. Further to this, the delegating style goes some way to facilitating maximum flexibility in which individuals choose to perform a given task.

Directing

Directing a paramedic's actions typically involves the complete *taking over* of patient care in a challenging or difficult situation. By applying this very intrusive style, a leader is able to utilize specific theoretical knowledge and clinical experience to enable appropriate, safe and accountable patient care.

A leader who engages in this style tends to establish quick and dynamic goals for the working environment as well as for the individuals under their remit. Simultaneously, the paramedics themselves continue to possess some scope for negotiated autonomy as to which skills are used to achieve their own ultimate patient care goals (Swansburg 2002). As case study 2.1 shows, care must be taken with this approach, do not ignore the need for excellent communication skills, so that all around you understand your decision-making. Obviously, in some circumstances, time is of the essence and patients' welfare comes before the feelings of your colleagues. If this does occur, a good clinical leader will make an effort to revisit the situation with the colleagues involved and explain their actions, if there was not initially time to do so.

Reflection: points to consider

Consider the examples of these styles from your own experience of whatever level or capacity of paramedic or role you currently undertake or have undertaken and match them to clinical profiles.

At this stage it should be noted that it is not just about having one particular style. As stated previously, it is more a matter of being able to adapt to the circumstances in a dynamic and ever changing environment. Maybe instead of just considering the need to learn how to apply one style, a good leader first needs to look at their own personal characteristics and see whether they have specific traits which tell them what type of leader they might be. There is a risk that they may be misguided in their judgement. Some personality characteristics such as determination, mindfulness and consideration are common to many people and should be further studied in more depth. These characteristics are generic but also specific to paramedics by means of their application to practice.

Self-evaluation exercise

Complete the leader/follower questionnaire and the abridged Myer-Briggs Personality Trait questions on pages 19–27 of Barr and Dowding's (2012) book, *Leadership in Health Care*. This will provide you with insight about some of the aspects of leadership that you may find easier than others. This self-awareness should enable you to understand more about your relationships with colleagues and areas of your leadership style that you may wish to focus on and develop in the future.

Further to this, a good leader has the ability to recognize value in the things that those around them do or have the potential to do; as a result of this recognition, they will continue to be willing to invest further time and effort in them.

Reflection: points to consider

Consider a leader you know who claims to have an 'open door' policy, think about that listening leader and how they are perceived by others. Who is the leader who is always there for you to talk to after that 'bad job'? Is it the same individual?

A good leader has the ability to share knowledge with those around them who need it or may benefit from it. Knowledge should not necessarily be seen as power, as Sir Francis Bacon once famously stated (Quotations Page 2013), the true power comes from how that knowledge is applied. There is a cadre of leaders who appear determined to withhold knowledge and information seemingly unnecessarily, but surely the more information that is made available, then (as a unit) strength and efficiency are improved, symbiotically benefitting the leader themselves in a 360° fashion.

Link to Chapter 3, for more information on organizational culture and power relations.

Leaders and power

Leaders who go some way to use their influence and power to benefit others are seen in a positive light. A good leader is just as interested in having a positive influence on their staff's development as they are in developing their own portfolio. This by no means detracts from the importance of their own personal development. On the contrary, they should lead by example, but effective leadership does not remove the desire to assist paramedics from the desire to be the best they themselves can be. There are always ways to consider self and others together. Failure of the leader to engage in their own development may mean that they become de-skilled and maybe even clinically incompetent. They need to be relied upon for their professionalism and their ability to complete the same tasks that they are asking their staff to perform.

Reflection: points to consider

What about success? Do you think that your leader should celebrate your success, even if it is greater than theirs? Surely they should not be concerned when others are successful?; they should be comfortable enough with their own successes not to feel destabilized. There may be realization that some staff have the potential to develop beyond the scope of their leader's domain, but this should not be seen as a threat.

One of the responsibilities that comes with leading is the service and development of those around you and the expectation that you will receive nothing back in return except a sense of achievement. Personal life-long learning and the implementation of what is learnt in practice (for the good of all) should be reward enough. Having others place value on the paramedics that are led means that the leader remains relatively valuable too, as well as accessible, personally approachable, and, more importantly, professionally accountable. They do not marginalize themselves away from people, regardless of the levels of responsibility that they have attained; they are more likely to ask for the views of their peers regarding the decisions that need to be made, and therefore this makes the decisions more positively viewed.

A sense of vision

And what of the future? A good leader should have vision as one of their characteristics. What is around the corner for them, their team and the organization for which they work? They should always be thinking beyond the here and now and asking what opportunities or challenges may present themselves next. The nature of the NHS means constant change. A good leader will keep abreast of new emerging ideas, and themes within healthcare that can be translated to the ambulance service.

For example, the 111 service has the potential to create more work for GP services. It has been widely reported that GP services are struggling to cope with the workload, and so is there a role for a paramedic working alongside GPs, or as part of a multi-professional team? This already occurs in some areas of the country, but a wider national approach may be required to meet the government's primary care agenda. There are two common threats to a leader, first, not envisaging the future, and, second, not being willing to encourage, promote and accept change, growth and healthy development of those around them.

Reflection: points to consider

What about a leader's personality and character? Do you want them to be above reproach, to work and succeed to the highest standards, to be *knowledgeable* on all issues when needed, to be *skilful* in their patient care and to conduct themselves in a *professional* manner, whether it is operationally or during their managerial duties?

Modern leadership theories

The NHS Leadership Academy (2013) asks us to consider a number of questions in order to make sense of the modern theories that support being a good contemporary paramedic leader.

What is leadership and who can do it?

First, it is encouraged that we understand what leadership truly is. We should look upon it as an entity that is not restricted to those who have job titles which are defined as managerial or supervisory, or even the traditionally recognized clinical leadership roles. They encourage all healthcare professionals, paramedics included, to recognize that the most successful leadership theories are the ones that possess shared responsibility for success within an organization.

Further questioning by the modern leader encourages analysis of who exactly can or should be a leader. There are theories which now suggest that acts of leadership come from all levels and grades within organizations. Emphasis is placed on the responsibility of staff to promote appropriate professional behaviours, to ensure staff contribution to the overall process, and also to develop and empower leadership capacity across the grades.

Shared and distributed leadership

A further contemporary theory in use is that of shared and distributed leadership. This model of leadership is particularly appropriate where complex tasks and highly interdependent roles are involved. A charismatic leader usually takes over a situation and establishes new goals and expectations (Spillane 2008). This is a familiar circumstance for paramedics in pre-hospital care and so it is worthwhile discussing this style. It is important to note that charisma is not an essential leadership characteristic (Barr and Dowding 2012). Leaders do not necessarily need charisma, but as humans we are drawn towards people who exude the personality characteristics that we refer to as charisma. Indeed, historically charismatic figures have not always been kind, but have managed to get vast numbers of people to follow their commands, such as Adolf Hitler. It is quite rightly accepted by many that not everyone is cut out to be a leader, but all grades of clinician can make vital contributions to the overall process by using the behaviours highlighted by the domains of the Leadership Framework presented in Box 2.1.

Link to Chapter 1 for the full Clinical Leadership Competency Framework.

Box 2.1   Domains of the Leadership Framework for those delivering the service

- Demonstrating personal qualities.
- Working with others.

- Managing services.
- Improving services.
- Setting direction.

Source: Leadership Academy (2011).

The Healthcare Leadership Model (2013) has a similar focus, but uses different terminology, such as 'engaging the team', as opposed to 'working with others'. Additional dimensions are more patient care and being organizationally focused, such as 'leading with care', 'evaluating information', 'holding to account' and 'influencing for results' being the ones that are very different to the previous Framework. The titles of these dimensions reflect the key findings and subsequent recommendations of the Francis Report. They are explained in more detail in the NHS Leadership Academy document.

Self-evaluation exercise

If you are a *junior member of staff*, the Leadership Academy recommends working through their Self-Assessment tool. It can be accessed through the following link: http://www.leadershipacademy.nhs.uk/discover/leadership-framework-self-assessment-tool/. This will enable you to examine your own personal characteristics and compare them with the domains of the Leadership Framework and the CLCF to identify areas where you excel and areas you can focus upon to improve your leadership potential.

For *leaders at stages 3 and 4* of the Leadership Framework (middle managers and above), the Leadership Framework (LF) 360° tool is recommended. It reflects the seven domains of the Leadership Framework. Staff who may benefit from undertaking the LF 360° might be:

- looking for further information on their leadership behaviours;
- wanting to benchmark their leadership performance against others;
- seeking to understand the impact of their behaviour on others;
- looking to draw up personal development plans.

This can be accessed at: http://www.leadershipacademy.nhs.uk/discover/leadership-framework-360-feedback-tool/. The tool will be updated to reflect the new Leadership Framework, once it is finalized and published, the website carries this additional note.

Stepping outside of the traditionally accepted theories, there are further modern interpretations to be considered. It is believed that leadership is an emerging social phenomenon in paramedic practice, a process that builds on a relationship within a peer group (Bolden and Gosling 2006; Woollard 2012). A further example of modern theory suggested by Goffee and Jones (2006) is one of leadership authenticity. This example suggests that leaders are seen to be more effective when being true to their own design. It is suggested by the authors that authentic leadership theory is about *being yourself, but more and with skill!*

Returning to the traditional theories which are still applied to modern paramedicine, it can be seen that criticism could potentially be aimed at many aspects as they do not fully consider the diverse and dynamic nature of the paramedic leader's role.

Reflection: points to consider

Blake and Mouton's (Mind Tools) leadership grid takes the treatment of task orientation and people orientation and divides them into two independent dimensions. Look at this, is this really possible in the modern paramedic leader where human outcomes are at the forefront of many decisions made?

Path-goal theory

House's path-goal theory (House 1996) warns the leader not to rise above or position themselves with *power*; it instead reminds us all that our core role as leaders is to assist our subordinates in the defining of goals before assisting them to achieve these goals in an efficient and effective manner.

Transformational and transactional leadership theories

Other modern theories that are tried and tested and have proven track records are transformational and transactional leadership. Transformational leadership has a place in the modern paramedic leadership structure due to its encouragement of inspiration and motivation, its offer of intellectual stimulation, the proportion of idealized influence and its high levels of individual consideration. Transactional leadership, on the other hand, goes some way to empowering those who are reluctant to be led, offering reward as a result of responding to instruction. Spend some time looking at the characteristics of these types of leaders in Table 2.1.

The NHS Leadership Strategy and its implications for leaders

The NHS Leadership Strategy (2013) encourages a staged approach to its delivery. The most imperative element is that all plans developed and agreed

Table 2.1 Characteristics of transactional and transformational leaders

Transactional leaders	Transformational leaders
Are responsive to change	Are proactive
Are effective within set cultures	Are able to change culture by instilling new ideas
Are able to use reward and punishment to invoke change	Achieve goals by means of motivation and the empowerment of others
Are able to encourage self-interest	Encourage self-value in order to influence whole groups
Are aware of the link between effort and reward	Arouse emotions which motivates those they lead to act beyond their framework
Deal with present issues	Are proactive and form new expectations
Rely on standard forms of reward, punishment and sanction	Are distinguished by their capacity to inspire and provide intellectual stimulation/idealized influence
Motivate by setting goals and promising rewards for desired performance	Can create learning opportunities and stimulate problem solving
Depend on power to reinforce subordinates towards successful completion	Possess vision, rhetorical and management skills, and develop emotional bonds
	Motivate their teams to work for goals that go beyond self-interest

are strategic and, more importantly, place the care of patients at their core. In order for this to come to fruition, all leaders need to demonstrate that they are effective in four key areas:

- *Framing* which allows the leader to take account of culture, history and long-term underlying issues. It also enables the use of sound organizational theory in order to inform the development of strategy and identify best practice. Finally, framing allows the leader to identify the best options to deliver their Trust's vision.

- Developing a *consistent approach* to leadership for all, irrespective of profession, role or grade. A consistent approach can represent the standard for behaviours that staff can aspire to.

- *Implementing strategic plans* that can be translated into something that is workable and operational. Part of this relates to identifying risks and the critical factors for success. The identification of capabilities required to deliver a strategy is important as is the establishment of clear line of accountability to hold people to account. During implementation, a leader has to be able to respond quickly and decisively when circumstances demand it.

- *Embedding* any strategy is the final key area. Walking away post-implementation with the knowledge that the strategy will remain in place should be a good leader's goal. Those who are responsible for delivering strategic and operational plans should feel motivated and inspired to continue, as this will help them to overcome any obstacles and challenges, and to remain focused. Those leaders should continue to monitor and evaluate outcomes, and, where necessary, make adjustments to ensure the strategy's sustainability.

The NHS Leadership Strategy has to be deliverable at both a national and local level. It is the responsibility of paramedic leaders to go through the process described above. They need to ensure that they *make it fit* with their Trust's requirements and cultures, that where gaps exist, then solutions are developed, that positive and decisive implementation occurs and that the final stage of embedding is achieved to the highest of standards.

Accountability and engagement

Trust leaders should not attempt these four stages on their own, however. In order to receive the necessary support, there is a requirement for them to step outside of the traditional NHS managerial circles and look to other areas for help. It is suggested that if paramedic leaders do not start (or continue) to work in such a way to develop strategies with those around them, then there is a risk of catastrophic strategic failure. This is perceived as vital, so input from a number of sources is essential for the successful implementation of any strategy (Aladwani 2001). A further risk is one of accountability. Unless paramedic leaders begin to take a higher degree of responsibility for those whom they lead, they will start to be seen as vicariously accountable for *their* failings too. It is important to remember that a need exists for strong leaders to fully enable positive organizational cultures that embrace change and the broader leadership strategy.

Link to Chapter 8 for more detail on managing and leading change and Chapter 4 for more on organizational culture.

When a paramedic is given a senior leadership role within an organization, it is essential that they draw on a range of available information, learned knowledge and operational experience if they are to engage in the strategy fully and promote it. There is a need to take into account cultural differences, organizational history, and the potential for long-term underlying issues. If this is achieved, then the paramedic leader will be in a stronger position to fully develop the strategy using best practice and all of the strategic options available to deliver their organization's ultimate vision. Further to this, paramedic leadership requires engagement with Trust colleagues and those who are in similar positions in regulatory or advisory capacities such as the

Health and Care Professions Council (HCPC) or the College of Paramedics. This engagement will help to further develop strategy by formulating plans to meet the organizational vision and attempt to understand their aims and motivators to develop sustainability. The creation of challenging and simultaneously realistic strategic plans is more likely to lead to achievement if the perspectives of others (including non-paramedics) are taken into consideration. Plans are more likely to be less risky and more certain to succeed on this basis. A strong paramedic leader has skills to implement a strategy that has been well developed. They are organized, clinically focused and able carry some of their Trust's risks so that they can fully implement the strategy. Translating that strategy into deliverable plans in the Trust can be challenging, but it is the key to success. Translation will include the identification of staff requirements to deliver the strategy and offering clear lines of accountability for that delivery, fully embedding and achieving the strategy.

For the strategy to be fully embedded, a paramedic leader has to be supportive and inspirational. They may not be directly responsible for the operationalization of plans, but they can assist and advise with the removal of obstacles to success. The creation of a professional leadership culture that embraces the views of others in order to support and promote strategic change in the modern pre-hospital environment can only be seen as positive. A transparent, trust-based approach, with open discussions encouraged, will facilitate the evaluation of pre-set strategic outcomes, and allow adjustments where needed, in order to sustain longevity.

Link to Chapter 8 for more on managing change and barriers to successful implementation of plans.

The true links between theory and practice

It is important for paramedics to examine the process of leadership, focusing on its application to what you do on a day-to-day basis. From the more historical theories through to the modern thinking, principles and concepts need to be fully understood. Focus needs to be maintained by a good leader on *real-world* circumstances and present-day application. Further to this is the need for the differences between managers and leaders to be identified in practice while simultaneously understanding why those differences are so important to the health of any organization or Ambulance Trust.

Self-evaluation exercise

Make a list under each heading of what you think the characteristics of a manager and a leader should be.

Role/characteristics of manager	Role/characteristics of leader

- Did you find this easy?
- Were there some 'roles' or 'characteristics' where the boundaries between leader and manager became blurred?
- Can you describe the differences between leaders and managers to a colleague?
- If not, then consider doing some more reading (see the suggested reading list at the end of this chapter for full references): Barr and Dowding (2012), pages 8–11; Gopee and Galloway (2009), pages 47–9, and Northouse (2013), pages 12–15.

To create realistic true links to practice, leadership theories consider the need for the involvement of teams and their development, motivation and manageability. This has to include heightened levels of collaboration and respect, whereupon in any given case or situation the paramedic leader can gather, consolidate, share, and cherish the views of their followers, and therefore reach joint goals with limited conflict by using evidence-based approaches. This did not happen in case study 2.1. There is more to making leadership decisions real than mere evidence, though, there are the softer considerations to be made, such as moral dilemma and ethical practice. All decisions made have to integrate personal, social, and corporate responsibility and one way of achieving this is by improving the leader's methods of communicating. Oral communication or written words (whether to individuals or groups) need to be clear, concise, well organized, and supported by relevant media for the specific circumstance.

Link to Chapter 9 for more information on conflict management and Chapter 6 for more on team working and group dynamics.

Motivation

Identifying motivation in practice can be difficult for a paramedic leader as many leadership circumstances involve change which can be unpopular with the workforce. In order to find the right motivators, it is suggested that the identification of workplace commitment is key. This will allow the incorporation of leadership influence and power needed to motivate all parties involved. This identification is going to require some research though, not something that many in the pre-hospital care setting are familiar with as yet. All organizations have a requirement to be able to evaluate and defend their actions and apply appropriate techniques, but not many leaders have the skills to perform true research, statistically analyse findings or defend their actions using real evidence yet, perhaps some further development in this area is needed?

> **Link to Chapter 8 for more on managing change successfully.**

The most positive characteristic of many paramedic leaders is their knowledge and understanding of the profession. Many can demonstrate that they are competent in the identification and integration of the various operational and clinical concepts, numerous theoretical perspectives and multiple historical trends, and this makes them key figures in the field of contemporary healthcare leadership. They need to be, because they need to fully evaluate the impact of change before applying the appropriate change models to make those changes a success. Many theories are used by leaders but it is important to try and identify what they look like in practice so that paramedics can see whether those theories are fit for purpose. In Table 2.2 are a few examples adapted from brighthub.com, study them (and their methods and achievements) closer.

Reflection: points to consider

Spend some time considering the modern Ambulance Trust structure and what responsibilities in terms of leadership each person has. Are different styles needed by those different leaders? Does Rosa Parks have to become Donald Trump as she develops through her career, finally ending up as Walt Disney?

Table 2.2 Well-known historical leaders and their perceived leadership style

Theory/Style	Leader
Charismatic	Winston Churchill
Participative	Donald Trump
Collaborative	Dwight Eisenhower
Transactional	Charles de Gaulle
Transformational	Walt Disney
Quiet	Rosa Parks
Servant	Mahatma Gandhi

Source: www.brighthub.com.

Conclusion

Modern paramedic leaders recognize that there are multiple characteristics that make them fit to lead, but what is not always accepted is the means by which we can encourage characteristics that are not present. Leaders do not have to be one person or another, they do not need to have one particular skill set. They need to have multiple personalities and be adaptable! While it can appear relatively easy to learn how to lead, there is definitely a tacit, in-built, unspoken requirement for those with positions of responsibility to have a natural ability on which to build the skills in the first instance. Leadership strategies such as those created by the modern NHS Trusts offer guidance and overarching structures to all, but the actual realistic delivery of the principles of any strategy comes down to high standards of leadership every time. Most Ambulance Trusts now have a clinical leadership structure in place in their emergency service. These structures include: student paramedics, paramedics, Specialist paramedics; Advanced paramedics and Consultant paramedics. It is essential that there is recognition at all levels that the responsibility to lead belongs to everybody in that structure, and that numerous characteristics will be needed by all.

Chapter key points

- Many characteristics which used to be perceived as strong, positive traits are now being challenged as outdated.
- The NHS Leadership Strategy was created in order to deliver leadership in a more scientific manner.
- The most successful paramedic leaders are the ones who are able to adapt their style to any given situation.
- A good leader has the ability to share knowledge with those around them who need it or may benefit from it.
- A good leader should have vision as one of their characteristics.
- The most imperative element is that all plans developed and agreed are strategic and, more importantly, place the care of patients at their core.
- Unless paramedic leaders begin to take a higher degree of responsibility for those whom they lead, they will start to be seen as vicariously accountable for their failings too.
- To create realistic true links to practice, leadership theories consider the need for the involvement of teams and their development, motivation and manageability.
- Identifying motivation in practice can be difficult for a paramedic leader as many leadership circumstances involve change which can be unpopular with the workforce.

- Leadership strategies such as those created by the modern NHS Trusts offer guidance and overarching structures to all, but the actual realistic delivery of the principles of any strategy comes down to high standards of leadership every time.

References

Aladwani, A.M. (2001) Change management strategies for successful ERP implementation, *Business Process Management Journal*, 7(3): 266–75.

Barr, J. and Dowding, L (2012) *Leadership in Health Care*. London: Sage.

Bolden, R. and Gosling, J. (2006) Leadership competencies: time to change the tune? *Leadership*, 2: 147.

Brighthub (2013) Available at: http://www.brighthub.com/ (accessed April 2013).

Donald Walters, J. (2000) *Art of Supportive Leadership*. London: Crystal Clarity.

Goffee, R. and Jones, G. (2006) *Why Should Anyone Be Led by You?: What It Takes to Be an Authentic Leader*. Boston: Harvard Business School Press.

Goldsmith, M. and Lyons, L.S. (2006) *Coaching for Leadership*, 2nd edn. London: Wiley.

Health Knowledge (2013) Available at: http://www.healthknowledge.org.uk/public-health-textbook/organisation-management/5a-understanding-itd/leadership-delegation (accessed May 2013).

House, R.J. (1996) Path-goal theory of leadership: lessons, legacy, and a reformulated theory, *The Leadership Quarterly*, 7(3): 323–52.

Leadership Academy (2011) *Leadership Framework*. Coventry: NHS Institute for Innovation and Improvement.

Leadership Academy (2012) Discover the Leadership Framework. Available at: http://www.leadershipacademy.nhs.uk/discover/leadership-framework/ (accessed January 2013).

Leadership Academy (2013) *Healthcare Leadership Model: The Nine Dimensions of Leadership Behaviour*. Version 1.0. Leeds: NHS Leadership Academy. Available at: www.leadershipacademy.nhs.uk/leadershipmodel (accessed 26 November 2013).

Mind Tools (2013) Available at: http://www.mindtools.com/pages/article/newLDR_73.htm (accessed February 2013).

NHS Change Model (2013) Available at: http://www.changemodel.nhs.uk/pg/groups/12195 (accessed May 2013).

Quotations Page (2013) Available at: http://www.quotationspage.com/quotes/Sir_Francis_Bacon (accessed December 2012).

Spillane, J.P. (2008) Distributed leadership, *The Educational Forum*, 69(2): 143–50.

Swansburg, R.C. (2002) *Introduction to Management and Leadership for Nurse Managers*, 3rd edn. London: Jones and Bartlett.

Woollard, M. (2012) The role of the paramedic practitioner in the UK, *Journal of Emergency Primary Health Care*, 4(1).

Suggested reading

Barr, J. and Dowding, L (2012) *Leadership in Health Care*. London: Sage. Chapters 2 and 4.

Gopee, N. and Galloway, J. (2009) *Leadership and Management in Healthcare*. London: Sage. Chapters 3 and 4.

NHS (2009a) *Clinical Leadership in the Ambulance Service Report*. London: NHS. Available at: www.wmas.nhs.uk.

NHS (2009b) *Future Leaders Study: The Leadership Capabilities and Capacities of Ambulance Services*. London: NHS. Available at: www.wmas.nhs.uk.

Northouse, P.G. (2013) *Leadership: Theory and Practice*, 6th edn. London: Sage.

Taylor, J. and Armitage, E. (2012) Leadership within the ambulance service: rhetoric or reality? *Journal of Paramedic Practice*, 4(8): 443–7.

Useful website

The NHS Leadership Academy: delivering the strategy http://www.leadershipacademy.nhs.uk/.

3 Clinical leadership in the National Health Service
Implications for paramedics

Linda Nelson and Mel Newton

In this chapter

- Introduction
- Clinical leadership
- Foundations for clinical leadership
- The link between leadership and power
- Leadership development
- Future direction
- The Clinical Leadership Competency Framework in action
- Conclusion
- Chapter key points
- References
- Useful websites

Introduction

The aim of this chapter is to explore clinical leadership in the National Health Service (NHS) and the drivers for leadership development by providing a historical perspective, a discussion about current clinical leadership, and looking to the future. The NHS clinical leadership momentum has developed over the past 20 years and to understand the change in philosophy, it is important to set it in context. Therefore, it should be acknowledged that serious events such as the Bristol Inquiry informed practices at that time, and today the Francis Inquiry is driving changes in service delivery. After looking back to see the context for clinical leadership, the link between power and leadership will be examined so that some application to practice can be considered. The chapter will refer to the Leadership Framework and encourage you to think about your role as a clinical leader within your organization and the wider NHS, as 'it is the responsibility of all staff to demonstrate appropriate behaviours, in seeking to contribute to the leadership process and to develop and empower the leadership capacity of colleagues' (NHS Institute 2009). Before you start reading this chapter, carry out the following activities.

Reflection: points to consider

- What does the term *clinical leadership* mean to you?
- Do you think you are a *clinical leader* and, if so, why?
- If you think you are not a *clinical leader*, why not?

The current status for leadership will now be explored and the framework for leadership is discussed. The underpinning leadership development will be reviewed and a possible insight into the future of clinical leadership is presented.

Clinical leadership

The expression *clinical leadership* may seem to be a clear and obvious concept in today's National Health Service (NHS) language. Most people would have some understanding of what clinical leadership means and who the clinical leaders might be. This has not always been the case, a look back at the history of the NHS will show how this nebulous concept has emerged and it is interesting to explore the foundations of the term. The aim here is to review the historical traditions and understand the way that clinical leadership has developed into the concept as we now understand it.

Foundations for clinical leadership

So why did clinical leadership emerge and what was the previous situation? According to McSherry et al. (2010), the political drivers for leadership development include a plethora of Department of Health documents published between 1999 and 2009, as detailed in Box 3.1, should you wish to read more detail.

Box 3.1   Department of Health documents 1999–2004, relevant to clinical leadership

1999	*Making a Difference*
2000	*National Health Service (NHS) Plan*
2000	*Meeting the Challenge*
2001	*NHS Action Plan Guide*

2001	*Working Together, Learning Together*
2001	*Making the Change*
2002	*Shifting the Balance of Power: The Next Steps*
2002	*Managing for Excellence*
2004	*NHS Improvement Plan*
2004	*National Standards, Local Action*
2004	*In Social Care: Leadership and Management Strategy for Social Care.*

In 2005, *Taking Health Care to the Patient* made a number of recommendations but specifically highlighted the need for leadership across a range of specialities. One of the final recommendations highlights the importance of clinical leadership: 'there should be improved opportunity for career progression, with scope for ambulance professionals to become clinical leaders'. More recently, the Operating Framework for the NHS in England (DH 2009) outlined the commitment to introduce talent and leadership plans at the regional and local levels. Indeed, effective clinical leadership was identified as central to the continuing development of the NHS, as long ago as 2001: 'Anyone working in the NHS, regardless of their position, grade, qualification or place of work, may be a leader or agent of change and improvement' (DH 2001: 52).

The link between clinical leadership and managing change in the NHS has been explicit. Moving forward in time, the Darzi Report (2008) was significant in so far that it emphasized development of high quality leadership by all clinicians, a point made explicit in Chapter 2 of this book. Traditionally in ambulance services, clinical leadership has been the primary role of the medical director and many of the doctors who fulfil the role come from a trauma or acute care background. However, the ambulance service has changed over the years with fewer patients being transported to hospitals. Paramedics are developing clinical decision-making skills to assess, treat and appropriately manage patients at home or refer them to other specialists and outside agencies, as exemplified in case study 3.1. Consequently, the change in service delivery, allied with the additional demands of academic progression and developing the professionalization of the paramedic, has led to the greater need to identify and nurture clinical leadership within the ambulance service (NHS Ambulance Chief Executive Group 2009). Therefore, appropriately trained leaders such as consultant paramedics have provided a wealth of knowledge and experience to influence future developments (Marsh 2009: 1), such as the role of paramedic practitioner (PP). As case study 3.1 demonstrates, clinical leadership is (and should be) at the grass roots of the ambulance service, and is not always (or should not be) *top down* in its approach. This holistic 'gold standard' care depends on the paramedic first on scene, considering the referral pathways and demonstrating clinical leadership by making the appropriate referral, with the best interests of the patient in mind. Without this referral to the PP, Joan's experience might have been very different.

Case study 3.1

A double-staffed vehicle (DSV) is mobilized to attend a call from a home address where an elderly patient has fallen. On arrival and following thorough assessment, the paramedic identifies the only injury to Joan is a pre-tibial laceration, which requires cleaning, steri-strip application and dressing, but this all takes quite a lot of time.

Prior to the introduction of paramedic practitioners into the Trust, the crew would have had very little choice but to take the lady to the nearest Emergency Department (ED) for treatment. While this would be an appropriate use of services, as it was an accident, it would mean potentially a long wait in the ED for Joan, exposure to viruses and bacteria there and the expense of getting her own way home after treatment.

The insightful paramedic contacts the referral desk within the Ambulance Trust and discusses Joan's injury with a paramedic practitioner, who agrees that Joan is an ideal candidate for referral to the ambulance paramedic practitioner (PP). The DMV crew apply a simple dressing to Joan's leg and inform her of the service provided by the PP, and the expected length of wait and obtain her consent for this course of action. Joan is duly referred.

The PP arrives, assesses, treats Joan's injury and during discussion also completes a social assessment to establish if there is a need for further social service input. The PP contacts Joan's GP surgery and makes a referral to the District Nurse, requesting a visit in two days time to re-assess and dress the wound. Joan is thoroughly satisfied with the treatment from the ambulance service, in fact, she is delighted that she has not had to leave her own home at all. She has had the opportunity to speak to some 'lovely people' and learnt that paramedics do not always 'whisk you off to hospital'.

The NHS Plan (2000) took the view that leadership must be evident at all levels of the NHS by both clinical and non-clinical staff, if improvements in care and efficiency were to be achieved. As can be seen by case study 3.1, this vision is coming to fruition in some ambulance services, particularly with improved education and subsequent role development. According to McSherry et al. (2010), this is a different approach from previous directives in that this plan recognized that an authoritarian approach would not facilitate effective change and development. Furthermore, Goodwin (2003) makes the distinction between using a leadership strategy as opposed to a managerial approach for Chief Executive or strategic level staff. He suggests that while a managerial approach based upon hierarchical position might be sufficient to effect a change in practice, a personal leadership style is more likely to produce a sustainable and longer-lasting outcome. The impact that a person has will be greater than the impact that a positional title may have.

The link between leadership and power

With this in mind, it is important to understand how change has been implemented in the NHS over time and how power has developed. Traditionally, the NHS implemented change using a variety of power strategies. The use of *reward power* refers to rewarding staff for compliance, for example, remuneration, awards, compliments, praise and social recognition. The long-term service awards reflect this respect for compliance and ensure that staff work within defined parameters. Members of staff who have worked for the NHS for a number of years are often held in high regard. Frequently the NHS is now accused of using *coercive power* which is grounded in fear. Examples of this can be seen in the threat of demotion, unwanted transfer to another department, withholding resources, loss of bonus payments, or threat of redundancy. The implication is that staff should not challenge the status quo and that compliance is expected. In the event of serious untoward incidents, staff report that they did not feel that they could raise concerns about professional practice by colleagues, especially if the colleague is perceived to be senior to them. *Legitimate power* is based upon authority to give instructions and again relies on a hierarchy structure. New activities procedures, policies, systems or strategies are imposed on the organization from a top-down perspective. In this situation the managers will be perceived to hold the power within the organization. By way of contrast, *expert power* is based upon knowledge and information. External consultants, internal specialists or well-informed senior managers might be seen to be the influencers here. Staff will defer to the clinical experts, regardless of positional power or length of service in the organization. *Information power* is used by people who have the ability to access non-public knowledge through personal connections. For example, secretaries to senior executives may be privy to sensitive information that is not available to others in the organization working at the same level. A similar classification might be *affiliation power*, where power is borrowed from a more genuine authority by association, for example, the personal assistant to the chief executive. This may be implicitly or explicitly threatening the direct involvement of the associated authority. *Referent power* depends on people's needs for leadership, inspiration and acceptance. Personal characteristics such as charisma, reciprocal identification (friendship), mutual interests, and collective perspectives are seen to be important.

Self-evaluation exercise

Think about cardio-pulmonary resuscitation and your varied experiences of it. Think about and answer the following questions:

- When you attend calls that involve cardiac arrest and cardio-pulmonary resuscitation, who leads the resuscitation?
- Is the answer to this question dependent on who is present at the time, or do you think the paramedic who is present from the beginning should maintain the leadership role?

- What if a more experienced, qualified paramedic arrives 15 minutes after you do, what then?
- Does the resuscitation lead paramedic need a *hands-on* role, or should they not touch the patient – leading from a distance?
- Referring to the different types of power explained in this chapter, which are applicable and why?

Of course, there are different care settings and organizational differences and contexts that must be considered. The Director of Operations, clinical profile 8, explains that she 'leads a team of approximately 2,400' and one of her core responsibilities is to ensure 'the professional leadership and management of all clinical operational staff'. This would be in direct contrast to a service provided by social services for young adults with Learning Disabilities in a residential setting. Here, the equivalent of Director of Operations, the 'care manager', would have a much smaller team and the role and responsibilities would reflect this. The type and style of leadership will be different, depending on the role and position the person has in the overall organization. The leadership style will also be influenced by the person taking the leadership role. Situational leadership as a type of leadership has been well documented. Indeed, clinical leaders should have an ability to adapt a personal leadership style to suit a particularly clinical context or setting.

Reflection: points to consider

- Think about your organization, can you identify different types of power associated with the different roles people have in it?
- How is power recognized and rewarded in your organization?
- What is the link between power and leadership?
- What is the link between power and management?

Leadership development

In the early part of the new millennium, the concept of transformational leadership dominated the leadership development programmes and was seen to place the importance of interpersonal and influencing skills at the heart of change for the NHS. Indeed, the transformational leadership model was used to inform the leadership development programme, Leading Empowering Organizations (LEO). It was thought that because nurses deliver 80 per cent of all healthcare, they should play a critical role in implementing the new NHS (Millward and Bryan 2005). The Royal College of Nursing developed a National Nursing Leadership Programme which also worked on the principle that clinical leadership was necessary at the supervisory level of the organization. The clinical grades F and G were targeted as being the key groups of staff ripe to be developed as clinical leaders.

Moving to the future, it is worth looking at the Francis Inquiry Report (2013) to understand the direction for leadership development, following the shocking standards at Stafford. The report suggests that '[the] common culture and values of the NHS must be applied at all levels of the organisation, but of particular importance is the example set by leaders'. The report calls for a leadership staff college to provide common professional training in leadership. It is suggested that an accreditation scheme enhancing eligibility for consideration for such roles will have the effect of promoting and researching best leadership practice. The report takes the view that the college should not be a *virtual organization* facilitating events but a physical presence that will serve the role of reinforcing the required culture through shared inter-professional learning. The leadership college will provide a common induction into the expectations of the NHS of those with leadership roles and responsibilities. Furthermore, a common code of ethics, standards and conduct for senior board-level healthcare leaders and managers should be produced and should be consistent with the common culture. It is recommended that non-compliance with the code could be grounds for considering a leader as not a fit and proper person to be in a leadership role.

In light of these Francis Inquiry Report recommendations, Chris Lake, Head of Professional Development at the Leadership Academy, in a conference speech on the 13th February 2013, described the levels of leadership development programmes that would be based upon the current NHS Institute Vanguard Programme which has two levels of leadership development. Emerging leaders and aspiring leaders at all levels and sectors of the NHS have evaluated it positively. It was suggested that leadership development programmes would be co-ordinated by the Leadership Academy and would extend to the Chief Executive Officer (CEO) level of development.

Self-evaluation exercise

Go to www.leadershipacademy.nhs.uk to find the Healthcare Leadership Model (version 1.0). Use the model to self-assess your leadership behaviours as suggested. The worksheet below can be used to record your results and you can identify a future date (perhaps 6 months' time) to identify any development in leadership skill.

Worksheet

Healthcare Leadership Model 2013

Name...

Date...

Review date...

	Essential	Proficient	Strong	Exemplary
Inspiring a shared purpose				
Leading with care				
Evaluating information				
Connecting our service				
Sharing the vision				
Engaging the team				
Holding to account				
Developing capability				
Influencing for results				

Notes

Future direction

When looking at the direction that policy drivers have taken with regard to leadership, it is interesting to note the subtle changes over time. While the NHS Plan and modernization agenda asked for strong leadership and high profile examples, this perspective has changed somewhat. Indeed, the leadership development programme called LEO emerged when the concept of clinical leadership was seen to play an important role in implementing the new NHS (DH 2002). The call for greater clinical roles (particularly nursing) to lead the process of change was at the forefront of policy (Millward and Bryan 2005). The notion of transformational leadership style to drive change was replaced by the idea that situational leadership is required. This suggests that the skills and qualities of the transformational leader might suit certain situations but a degree of flexibility was now required. Each clinical situation would require a different approach and a different skill set. This is certainly the case in the paramedic profession due to the wide variety of clinical situations that paramedics find themselves in, and caring for patients across the lifespan. This makes sense and clearly the change needed to improve patient care has to be context-appropriate. However, the message remains that one leader would be followed by the majority. The role of the leader still seems to be in line with hierarchical structures and management position. Indeed, the leadership framework is a good illustration of how this would work and embraces the message that all individuals have responsibility for clinical leadership that is context-relevant.

The Clinical Leadership Competency Framework in action

Case study 3.2

A community responder attends a cardiac arrest of a 58-year-old man at his home with his wife and two children (ages 16 and 24) present. Colleagues soon arrive, a paramedic crew. A solo responder, a critical care paramedic, is also on his way, estimated time of arrival 15 minutes. Resuscitation following Trust protocol is underway. The community responder is asked by the paramedics to care for the distressed family, obtain a patient history from the family, and take them to an adjacent room, while the paramedics continue resuscitation.

Fifteen minutes pass and the critical care paramedic (CCP) arrives, takes hand-over from both the community responder and the paramedics. The critical care paramedic reviews what has been carried out to date, talks through what everyone has done, reviews treatment, and the protocol. The paramedics continue with resuscitation while the CCP considers what the team can do next.

With reference to the core domains of the leadership framework (NHS Leadership Academy 2011b), detailed in Chapter 1 of this book, think about the domains in relation to case study 3.2 and the qualities the professional registrants demonstrate.

Both paramedics and the CCP exhibit domains 1 and 2, *Demonstrating personal qualities* and *Working with others*. Domain 3, *Managing services* applies, as it is focused on managing people and managing performance. Both paramedics demonstrated competence in this aspect of the domain, prior to and after the arrival of the CCP. While none of the employees were directly focused upon the success of the organization in which they work, they were directly focused on the patient's survival, which implicitly reflects their organization. Domain 4, *Setting direction*, can be discussed from an organizational perspective or from a patient-focused perspective, as is the focus in case study 3.2. The paramedics certainly did apply their knowledge and evidence base in order to make decisions for this patient and to evaluate the impact of their actions.

Domains 5 and 6 apply particularly but not exclusively to individuals in senior positional leadership roles. *Creating the vision* (domain 5) and

Delivering the strategy (domain 6) respectively, are generally regarded as organizational in nature. But without the paramedics who undertake the additional education and shoulder the responsibility to act in advanced roles, such as the CCP, the organizational vision would flounder and not fulfil the overall strategy.

Link to Chapter 2 for more theories of leadership.
Link to Chapter 4 for organizational effects on leadership.

Emotional intelligence

Looking to the future direction, the art of leadership is recognized as being integral to how a person implements change. The artful leader should be attuned to the undercurrents of emotion that pervade a group. Leadership credibility is achieved by the leader acting as a mirror to reflect back to the group its own experience (Goleman 1999). The impact of emotional intelligence with regards to effective leadership is well evidenced. In this way, differences between management and leadership positions can be identified. Goleman (1999) refers to the leadership competencies and identifies three main clusters. These include personal competencies such as achievement, self-confidence and commitment. He also suggests that influence, political awareness and empathy are imperative to successful leaders, while cognitive competencies include the ability to think strategically, seek information and apply conceptual thinking. Indeed, leadership demands that people's imagination is required to inspire them to move in a desired direction; it takes more than positional power to motivate and lead others. So where will the emotionally intelligent leader emerge and what will be their remit for the future?

Link to Chapter 8 for more information on managing change.

Bevan (2011) records key messages with regards to the future development of the NHS and uses the expression that we need to 'build leadership systems that are managerially loose but culturally tight'. This notion suggests that rather than relying upon a few top managers with a leadership responsibility, future direction means that control has to be relinquished and micro-management reduced. Bevan further suggests that collective action towards a different future with shared purpose is needed. As healthcare demands become increasingly more complex, an innovative approach to leadership is required; this is referred to as a *distributed system* and makes sense. Future leaders are likely to include service users and local government personnel, voluntary and independent sector leaders who will be called to action with a united sense of purpose around a common cause. This distributed leadership approach is about widening the pool of leaders in the system. The focus for the development of leadership talent is likely to change and, according to Beer (cited in Bevan 2011), the perspective will be that 'varieties of expertise are distributed across the many, rather than the few'. The use of a *call to action* methodology has been successful with examples such as the initiative around better care for people with dementia who had been prescribed anti-psychotic drugs.

With regard to large-scale change, Barlett and Ghoshal (cited in Bevan 2011) state that 'the leader's most basic role is to release the human spirit that makes initiative, creativity and entrepreneurship possible'. They go on to talk about the human passion based on the belief that there is a different and better way that is worth time and effort to strive for. They advocate the use of transformative narratives that draw on personal experiences and align with individual and collective values.

Partnership approach and range of leadership styles

It is recognized that it may not be one person leading a team. In fact, Quinn (2004) would suggest that the function of leadership is to produce more leaders, not followers. The notion of followership has been explored by Moiden (2003) and it can be suggested that the roles of leadership and followership should not be fixed but should be fluid and flexible. For example, a leader who leads from behind might agree to follow a different person with the necessary skills and competencies required for the task at hand. Should the paramedic always state a course of action or can it be more appropriate for a student paramedic to suggest a treatment plan?

While different skills and attributes will comprise a team, there are other considerations to take into account. Ham (2003) suggests that as professionals have a degree of control, politicians and managers need clinical staff to influence decision-making from a bottom-up perspective. While Ham (2003) refers to studies on medical clinicians, the principles hold true for all NHS clinical staff. He identified that the clinicians were unlikely to buy into a change unless the benefits for patients or the service were clearly evident.

Collaborative working and inter-professional approaches cannot be underestimated. Again the type and style of the multi-professional team will reflect the type of care setting. Recently developments have been made to include service users and carers in some operational team structures. Furthermore, it has been suggested that some service users should take a key leadership role in helping to shape service delivery. While this is evident in mental health services, the principles might be applied to other care and treatment services.

At an event in March 2013, Steve Fairman, Director of Business, Improvement and Research with the NHS Commissioning Board, shared his perspective on the future direction for leadership. He referred to the last ten years as having a management focus while the next ten years will need a leadership using a partnership approach. He suggested that while the past had leadership with limited styles, the future required a broad range of styles. While the past leadership centred around organizations, the new leadership would span across systems. With regard to the location, the past leaders were very much *in the room* and the future leadership will be much more virtual and *in the ether*. While the last ten years allowed leadership to be *in camera*, the leaders in the next ten years will be very much in public view. Fairman goes on to suggest that the previous leadership approach was to hit targets while the future direction will be more about continuous improvement. The quotation from David Lloyd George, used by Fairman (2013) 'about being ambitious but recognising that you can't take two steps over a gap', is a sound illustration of the *small steps* philosophy that could underpin large-scale change initiatives.

Conclusion

In conclusion, this chapter has outlined some of the drivers for clinical leadership and the political agenda influence has been identified. Links with power and management have been discussed and the role of clinical leadership for paramedics included. The future direction for clinical leadership with regard to large-scale change has been explored. The impact of the Francis Inquiry Report on the future direction for leadership development has been highlighted.

Chapter key points

- In essence, clinical leadership is about clinical staff at all levels being actively engaged in the continuous improvement of the quality and safety of patient services.
- A number of key national policy drivers have made numerous references to leadership as part of the core business of the NHS.
- Partnership working will be at the forefront of the NHS agenda in the coming years.
- NHS policies and drivers are applicable to the ambulance service and to the clinical leadership role of paramedics.
- Leadership skills will need to transcend the organizational boundaries we know today, ambulance service personnel will increasingly be required to work with other professionals.
- The NHS clinical leadership agenda has developed over time and a distributed model of leadership is now required.

References

Bevan, H. (2011) *Part 2, Leading Large-Scale Change: The Postscript.* London: NHS Institute for Innovation and Improvement.

Cameron, K.S., Quinn, R.E., Degraff, J. and Thakor, A.V. (2006) *Competing Values Leadership: Creating Value in Organizations.* Cheltenham: Edward Elgar Publishing.

College of Paramedics (2013) *Paramedic Curriculum Guidance*, 3rd edn. Bridgwater: College of Paramedics.

Covey, S.R. (2004) *The 7 Habits of Highly Effective People: Powerful Lessons in Personal Change.* London: Simon & Schuster.

Covey, S.R. (2005) *The 8th Habit: From Greatness to Effectiveness.* New York: Free Press.

Darzi Report (2008) *High Quality Care for All: NHS Next Stage Review Final Report.* London: Department of Health.

Department of Health (1999) *Making a Difference.* London: Department of Health.

Department of Health (2000a) *The NHS Plan.* London: Department of Health.

Department of Health (2000b) *Meeting the Challenge: A Strategy for the Allied Health Professions.* London: The Stationery Office.

Department of Health (2001a) *Making the Change: A Strategy for the Professions in Healthcare Science.* London: Department of Health

Department of Health (2001b) *Working Together, Learning Together.* London: Department of Health.

Department of Health (2002a) *Shifting the Balance of Power: The Next Steps.* London: Department of Health.

Department of Health (2002b) *Managing for Excellence in the NHS.* London: Department of Health.

Department of Health (2004a) *National Standards, Local Action: Health and Social Care Standards and Planning Framework 2005/06–2007/08.* London: Department of Health.

Department of Health (2004b) *Knowledge and Skills Framework.* London: Department of Health.

Department of Health (2005) *Taking Health Care to the Patient: Transforming NHS Ambulance Services.* London: Department of Health.

Department of Health (2009) *The Operating Framework for the NHS in England 2009/10.* London: Department of Health.

Department of Health (2013) *Report of the Mid Staffordshire NHS Foundation Trust Public Inquiry: Executive Summary* (The Francis Inquiry Report). London: TSO.

Edwards, G. (2002) Leadership: a qualified case for accreditation. *Training Journal*, June, pp. 20–1.

Fairman, S. (2013) Speech at the NHS Vanguard Programme Celebration Event, Mary Ward House, London, 20 March.

Goldsmith, M. and Reiter, M. (2006) *What Got You Here Won't Get You There: How Successful People Become Even More Successful.* New York: Hyperion.

Goleman, D. (1999) *Working with Emotional Intelligence.* London: Bloomsbury.

Goodwin, N. (2003) Making leadership work in today's NHS, *British Journal of Health Care Management*, 9(5): 179–81.

Graetz, F., Rimmer, M., Lawrence, A. and Smith, A. (2002) *Managing Organisational Change.* London: Wiley.

Grohar-Murray, M.E. and Dicroce, H.E. (2002) *Leadership and Management in Nursing*, 3rd edn. London: Pearson Education.

Ham, C. (2003) Improving the performance of health services: the role of clinical leadership, *The Lancet*, 361(9373): 1978–80.

Hayes, J. (2002) *The Theory and Practice of Change Management*. Basingstoke: Palgrave.

Health and Care Professions Council (2012) *Position Statement on the NHS Clinical Leadership Competency Framework (CLCF)*. London: HCPC.

Johnson, G. (2002) Keeping leadership simple: the executive summary approach, *Training Journal*, June, pp. 28–30.

Kouzes, J.M. and Posner, B.Z. (2002) *The Leadership Challenge*, 3rd edn. San Francisco: Jossey-Bass.

Lake, C. (2013) Paper presented at 'Aspiring Leaders to Leaders' Conference, NHS London, 13 February.

Little, S. (2008) *The Milkshake Moment: Overcoming Stupid Systems, Pointless Policies and Muddled Management to Realize Real Growth*. Hoboken, NJ: John Wiley & Sons.

Malone, B. (2002) Nurses offered bigger leadership roles, *Primary Care Partnerships*, 5: 1.

Mann, D. (2005) *Creating a Lean Culture: Tools to Sustain Lean Conversions*. New York: Productivity Press.

McSherry, M., Smith, L. and Kell, J. (2010) Leadership and change management, in R. McSherry and J. Warr (eds) *Implementing Excellence in Your Health Care Organisation*. Maidenhead: Open University Press.

Millward, L.J. and Bryan, K. (2005) *Clinical Leadership in Health Care: A Position Statement*. The Emerald Research Register, pp. xiii–xxv.

Moiden, N. (2002) Evolution of leadership in nursing, *Nursing Management*, 9(7): 20–5.

Moiden, N. (2003) A framework for leadership, *Nursing Management*, 9(10): 19–23.

NHS Ambulance Chief Executive Group (2009) *Report of the National Steering Group on Clinical Leadership in the Ambulance Service*. London: NHS.

NHS Institute for Innovation and Improvement (2005) *NHS Leadership Qualities Framework*. Available at: http://www.nhsleadershipqualities.nhs.uk (accessed 27 July 2013).

NHS Institute for Innovation and Improvement and Academy of Medical Royal Colleges (2009) *Shared Leadership Underpinning of the MCLF*. Coventry: NHS Institute for Innovation and Improvement.

NHS Leadership Academy (2011a) *Leadership Framework*. Coventry: NHS Institute for Innovation and Improvement.

NHS Leadership Academy (2011b) *Clinical Leadership Competency Framework*. Coventry: NHS Institute for Innovation and Improvement.

NHS Leadership Academy (2011c) *Guidance for Integrating the Clinical Leadership Competency Framework into Education and Training*. Coventry: NHS Institute for Innovation and Improvement.

NHS Leadership Academy (2013) *Healthcare Leadership Model: The Nine Dimensions of Leadership Behaviour*. Version 1.0. Leeds: NHS Leadership Academy. Available at: www.leadershipacademy.nhs.uk/leadershipmodel (accessed 26 November 2013).

Northouse, P.G. (2013) *Leadership Theory and Practice*, 6th edn. London: Sage.

Quinn, R. (2004) *Building the Bridge as You Walk on It: A Guide for Leading Change*. San Francisco: Jossey-Bass.

Seddon, J. (2005) *Freedom from Command and Control: Rethinking Management for Lean Service*. New York: Productivity Press.

Shapiro, A. (2004) *Creating Contagious Commitment: Applying the Tipping Point to Organisational Change.* North Carolina: Strategy Perspective.

Skills for Care (2004) *Leadership and Management: A Strategy for Social Care Workforce.* Available at: www.skillsforcare.org.uk (accessed 27 July 2013).

Useful websites

www.modernnhs.nhs.uk.
www.NHSLeadershipQualities.nhs.uk.
www.nursingleadership.org.uk.

4 Understanding the organization

Amanda Blaber

Introduction

The National Health Service (NHS) is generally referred to as a national *institution*. It is nonetheless an organization, albeit a huge, multi-faceted, complex one. Currently, the NHS serves 63.2 million people. The NHS employs more than 1.7 million people, in a range of roles, just under half are clinically qualified, including 39,780 general practitioners (GPs), 370,327 nurses, 18,687 ambulance staff and 105,711 hospital and community health service (HCHS) medical and dental staff. The NHS in England is the biggest part of the system by far, catering to a population of 53 million and employing more than 1.35 million people. The NHS in Scotland, Wales and Northern Ireland employs 153,427, 84,817 and 78,000 people respectively. The NHS cares for over 1 million patients every 36 hours.

NHS Choices website states that 'only the Chinese People's Liberation Army, the Wal-Mart supermarket chain and the Indian Railways directly employ more people'. This provides a sense of scale when thinking about the NHS as one organization (http://www.nhs.uk). As such a huge organization, control of local services has been devolved to regional levels for all types of care. There are currently 11 NHS Ambulance Trusts in England.

The NHS Ambulance (Foundation) Trusts in England form more geographically local organizations, albeit covering large diverse regions. This has not always been the case, as an exploration of the historical perspectives will explain. In order to understand your organization, it is important to explore the theory and reality of the concept of an organization. Structures of organizations vary and can have effects on the efficiency and effectiveness of the organization. Ambulance services are large, often complex organizations within the NHS. Organizations often have unique characteristics and cultures. All of the aforementioned will influence the experience of employees and patients in ambulance service organizations.

Historical perspectives of ambulance services as organizations

The history of health service development often influences the direction and future approaches to healthcare. To this day, the perception of the general public and indeed the expectations of the ambulance service are one of emergency response, caring for patients with serious illness, treatment and transportation of patients to hospital. Prior to the late 1960s, ambulance services were only used as a means of transport. Wide national variation existed in emergency techniques and technologies available. Education consisted of general first aid with the emphasis being on transportation of the casualty.

Newton (2012a) states that the major weaknesses in the ambulance service were identified by national reports of the late 1960s (Ministry of Health 1966; Ministry of Health, Scottish Home and Health Department 1967). These publications identified a lack of standardization across the UK. In 1963, 146 local authorities had control of ambulance services, instead of the regional control that we are familiar with today. Lack of resources, poorly equipped vehicles, poorly educated staff, poor pay, were some of the main problems. Lack of standardization of qualifications for both driving and attending staff was also identified. As a result, the 1960s publications are integral to the subsequent changes in ambulance services that took place through the 1970s and 1980s.

Reflection: points to consider

- Watch the 10-minute clip from the 1963 BBC *Panorama* programme which focuses on the ambulance services across the UK and discusses many of the points subsequently made in the Ministry of Health publications of the late 1960s. The link is: http://www.bbc.co.uk/archive/nhs/5161.shtml.

- Did the exposure of the problems lead to a government investigation and subsequent recommendations?

With the promise and reality of more resources, better equipped vehicles and the push towards more regional standardization, the focus in the 1970s and 1980s was on improving the standard of care for patients. This obviously required improved education and training for the attendants. Three key areas emerged: triage, emergency care and resuscitation. The focus on these three areas by pioneers, such as Larrey (Richardson 1974), Baskett (in the 1960s) and Chamberlain (in the 1970s and 1980s), has served ambulance service organizations well. These areas were the obvious weaknesses, considering the societal and political expectations of ambulance services during this era: to prioritize, provide life-saving care to sick people and transport them to the closest hospital facility.

Although the early pioneers' emergency focus was essential, it may have prevented earlier adaptation and diversification, in response to changing political, financial and societal developments (Newton 2012a, 2012b). This may be the case, but the paramedic profession had to take time to develop, create its own identity and become expert in the emergency care arena before it had the confidence and appropriately educated and skilled staff to successfully diversify. Today, we see paramedics undertaking in-depth physical and social assessment, prioritizing, referring to other agencies, taking patients to appropriate medical facilities (sometimes not the most local one) or treating the patient in their own home to prevent unnecessary transportation and hospitalization. This, of course, enables the government to meet their political agendas, but also provides a comprehensive and potentially diverse career structure for paramedics and many more alternatives than were available even in the 1990s. More importantly, these developments also contribute to a more satisfied patient, whose experience of the NHS has been one of seamless care by caring, knowledgeable and professional staff.

Ambulance services are generally creative, responsive organizations that are able to change to meet challenges and will be required to meet the health and social care service demands of the future. Such changes are also reflected in the ambulance organizations and their ability to respond to the NHS of the twenty-first century.

Link to the paramedic profiles and Chapter 1 for more detail on the varied roles and career development available to paramedics.

Uniqueness of ambulance services as organizations

Origins of ambulance service structure

The military association relating to the history of the ambulance service is well documented (Richardson 1974; Craggs and Blaber 2008; Newton 2012b). As an organization, the militia has a very hierarchical structure and chain of command. The ambulance service has historically also developed chains of command that are very formally structured, with clear boundaries. This is not unique to ambulance services, many other areas of the NHS are similar, but it is fair to say the ambulance service hierarchies have generally survived the vast changes that have affected other parts of the NHS for a number of years.

Occupational stress and sickness

Ambulance work is often unpredictable. As a result, paramedics and other ambulance personnel often work in chaotic and rapidly changing environments. The nature of work location (people's homes or streets) adds an element to the role that many other NHS employees do not experience. Mildenhall (2012) suggests all of the above contribute to occupational stress of ambulance clinicians. Sickness rates in the ambulance service are higher than the NHS as a whole (NAO 2011), but it is recognized there is a 60 per cent variation in sickness rates across the Ambulance Trusts in England. The National Audit Office state that there are cultural issues around short-term sickness (NAO 2011). Cultural issues may be organizational in nature (specific to certain organizations) or prevalent in certain professional groups (NAO 2011). In an attempt to explain such NHS variations, it is possible that Ambulance Trusts may have been understaffed, in respect of frontline paramedic staff, in recent years, possibly providing one reason for increased sickness rates. When compared to the rest of the NHS, ambulance services have seen a 15 per cent increase in staff numbers, compared to 7 per cent in qualified clinical staff across the NHS. The National Audit Office for the Department of Health (2011) states that the 15 per cent is not made up entirely of registered frontline staff in some Ambulance Trusts. As there is very limited UK research into such issues, assumptions and educated guesses are the only conclusions this chapter is able to provide.

Support networks

The uniqueness of the role of a paramedic has a potential effect on how employees work within the organization and how the organization may respond. Like other primary care NHS staff (health visitors, district nurses), paramedics either work in very small teams (as an ambulance crew) or are lone workers (critical care paramedics, paramedic practitioners, community care paramedics). The introduction of lone responders and geographical 'stand-by' points (primarily as a means to meet response target times) has reduced the opportunity for informal peer debrief, which is a valuable coping strategy identified by Mildenhall (2012).

This may link directly to staff sickness, but there is no UK research to substantiate this claim. NHS staff working in a more static working environment, such as a hospital ward, report more satisfaction and support in times of crisis from supervisors and managers, than paramedics do (Regehr and

Millar 2007). Mildenhall (2012) suggests the ambulatory nature of the work makes managerial support more difficult to facilitate, even though paramedics would welcome support, but were demoralized when it was promised and did not happen. Hence ambulance organizations need to adapt and develop communication and managerial strategies to overcome these difficulties and potentially damaging experiences for staff. Storey and Holti (2013) reinforce that staff well-being is an important element for leaders to achieve their full leadership potential.

Reflection: points to consider

- What support is available in your Ambulance Trust, should you require it?
- Who makes the decision that you may need support, or not?
- Is there a structured support system and clear guidance on how to access it?
- Is the support offered and provided by the Trust consistent?
- Or is it dependent on your line managers and their approach to leadership/management?

Gender and support networks

The gender difference between the ambulance service and other parts of the NHS is worth exploring. In 2012, 10.5 per cent of registered nurses and midwives were male (NMC 2012), compared to 69.1 per cent of registered paramedics being male (HCPC 2012). Female staff within the ambulance service constitute one-third of the workforce, and this is increasing year on year (Bendall, pers. comm. 2012; Lindenburg 2012). The construction of the workforce has an impact on coping strategies. Essex and Benz-Scott (2008) also note the number of years of service, in addition to gender, as having an impact on coping with stress in the ambulance service. Males tend to use less emotion and support networks (seeking social support and venting emotions) in comparison to females. In research by Prati et al. (2009), men described using avoidance coping (denial, self-distraction, behavioural disengagement and self-blame). Interestingly, there was no gender difference in respect of using humour as a coping strategy. The use of humour in emergency service work is an accepted part of the culture and role that people adopt while at work. It becomes part of who we are and for outsiders sometimes this can appear insensitive, inappropriate and, on occasions, unprofessional. When student paramedics are in the emergency care environment for the first time, this may be quite overwhelming and a challenge for them to understand and appreciate the role that humour plays in the everyday lives of emergency care workers. This research may indicate that though paramedics in Mildenhall's (2012) study would welcome support, if provided, it may not be readily accessed by many male paramedics. It could be that the findings indicate that clinicians want the reassurance (that if needed) assistance is there and that the organization cares about their employees. Prati, Palestini and Pietratoni (2009) identified that the avoidance coping strategies readily used by male emergency care workers are strongly correlated to burn-out, possibly providing a link to reasons for sickness. A closer examination of sickness statistics for UK Ambulance Trusts is needed. The elements for a new Leadership Model for the NHS (Storey and Holti 2013: 8) point to a potential new era where one element of the leadership strategy will be to 'listen to staff and respond to their voice, validate and engage with difficult or negative emotions evoked by the experience of delivering care, rather than suppress or deny them'. This is an attempt to motivate teams and individuals to work effectively. This will not happen unless an organization examines its own culture, structures and characteristics.

Characteristics of an organization

The NHS in England is subject to the politics of the governing political party of the UK. This steers the direction of the NHS for potentially short periods of time (5-year electoral cycles), though it can feel like an eternity when you are working with constant change and reform! To work within the NHS, you need to be mindful of the amount of change you will experience over the course of your career. The organization that first employs you will change in structure and culture over the years of your employment. Those of you who are employed by the ambulance service will have seen numerous changes, reforms and organizational restructures over the course of your employment. Many theorists have explored the nature of organizations, the reasons for change, the varieties of structures and the effect on employees. Some of their ideas and theories are explored in this section.

Why do organizations exist?

Marquis and Huston (2009) believe organizations are developed because more work can be accomplished by organizations than any one individual, working alone, can achieve. We all spend our lives as part of social, personal and professional organizations and constantly move between the roles we have in each organization. What is an organization?

> A social unit of people, systematically structured and managed to meet a need or to pursue collective goals on a continuing basis.
>   (www.businessdictionary.com/definition/organization.html)

The characteristics of an organization are summarized in Table 4.1. This table is only a summary and many more characteristics exist, some more prevalent depending on the organization. The characteristics explained in Table 4.1 are commonly discussed in the literature.

Table 4.1 Characteristics of organizations

Working as a group	Overcomes all the problems of working alone, i.e. time to achieve the task, e.g. crews of two people, or small teams.
Task-focused	Has been formed for a purpose – to get things accomplished, e.g. working groups to implement a new idea or evaluate clinically focused topic. Can be short or long term in focus.
Logical-rational based	Has ordered, logical processes, procedures and protocols. There is also concern to achieve the task to a set standard. Often has organizational set policies and procedures with quality assurance mechanisms.
Exchange based	People exchange with others and receive a mixture of benefits (financial, non-financial, psychological) from working. The organization receives time, effort, skills and commitment.
Improved productivity	Employees specialize in what they do and can combine their efforts with others. Additional roles often improve quality of care, e.g. community care paramedic/paramedic practitioner.
Quantitative more than qualitative focused	Achievements are usually more important than the quality of the relationships involved for the individual worker in getting tasks done. Organizations who strongly exhibit this characteristic are often more focused on the task.
Develops own identity, ethos and culture	This affects everyone who works within the organization. See case study 4.1.
Offers companionship	These can be simple or complex, but in many cases is a means to getting the task achieved in a timely, friendly manner.

Case Study 4.1

Phil is a 19-year old student paramedic, who has been at his first placement for 4 months. He has settled in well, feels he is part of the team and is really enjoying his placement. He is getting used to the culture of the station and to the banter of his co-workers. Phil's colleagues find him friendly, enthusiastic and describe him as 'settling in well'.

On station, Frank is usually the butt of most jokes. He is nearing retirement and has worked with most of his colleagues for many years. Phil has witnessed many jibes at Frank over the past four months and has laughed along with his colleagues.

On this occasion, Phil makes a joke at Frank's expense, involving calling him an *old timer*. The room falls silent and Phil is told in no uncertain terms that he has no right to make a joke about Frank, as he is not part of the team. He is told he is 'only a student' and has 'overstepped the mark' and has acted 'unprofessionally'.

Phil is devastated by this response, he thought he was part of the team, but it seems he was wrong.

Usually most organizations demonstrate each of the characteristics described in Table 4.1. Some characteristics will be more prevalent than others, depending on the type of business, structures and cultures within the organization. Case study 4.1 highlights one particular ambulance station, in terms of identity, ethos and culture. It may not reflect the whole organization, but impacts the behaviour of the staff working there. Who do you think is to blame for the situation Phil finds himself in? It is easy for employees to underestimate the strong culture and practice within their workplace. It may be intimidating for newcomers, who very often have to do their time, before they can express an opinion or let their guard down. Certainly the structure of the ambulance service (smaller location-based stations) contributes to the culture of individual stations. One Ambulance Trust may have many sub-cultures within it, these are often station based. Many Ambulance Trusts are restructuring the idea of smaller stations in favour of larger 'super-stations', regionally located. Storey and Holti (2013) advocate that organizations operate *meaningful design*, and address system problems by initiating new structures in order to focus on improving system performance. A consequence of this new structure might be reduction in the strength of sub-cultures.

Reflection: points to consider

Think about your organization, which of the characteristics mentioned in Table 4.1 would you say are more prevalent there?

What characteristics would you regard as priorities for your organization?

Structure of organizations

Marquis and Huston (2009) believe all organizations have a formal (visible and planned) structure and an informal (unplanned, often hidden) structure. In most Ambulance Trusts there is a well-defined, formal structure. Roles and functions are well defined and systematically arranged, with different people having differing roles, with rank and hierarchy being evident. However bureaucratic organizations are, they are dynamic, interactive and emotional, because people work within them. Ambulance Trusts are no different and, in many respects, can be considered more emotional because of the nature of the work and patient interactions, especially of paramedics and other emergency frontline workers.

The informal structure is usually social in nature with blurring or shifting lines of authority and accountability. As can be seen from Table 4.1, people are very much at the heart of any organization's characteristics and, as such, have the potential to influence the organization. Such networks exist in every organization, even if they are not officially recognized or acknowl-edged. These have the potential to be very powerful and should not be underestimated or ignored.

Link to Chapter 2 to explore leadership theory in more depth.

In order to develop an organizational structure Galbraith's (1977) 'Fit' model advocates remembering the five functions of an organization (see Box 4.1), as any change to organizational structure will affect the work of the organi-zation and its ability to work efficiently. The functions identified in Box 4.1 are not in any priority order, but a change to any of the functions will affect the equilibrium and function of the organization.

Box 4.1   The five functions of an organization (Galbraith 1977)

Work

Structure

People

Rewards

Information and decision- making e.g. IT, policies.

The nature of the work the organization does needs always to be central to any decision-making or changes within the organization. As Box 4.1 indi-cates, the structure needs to support the work the organization is involved in, as do the appropriately qualified staff who should be rewarded for the work that they do. Any organization also needs to consider the informa-tion required to make decisions so the organization works efficiently and effectively.

Types of organizational structures

There are several organizational structures commonly used in healthcare settings. The following are ones that may be seen in Ambulance Trusts, rather than hospital settings:

- organization pyramid or hierarchical vertical structure (tall or flat);

- complex matrix;

- parallel structure.

Reflection: points to consider

Take a look at your organizational structure, most Trusts will have a visual representation on their Intranet sites. Which of the types does it most closely represent?

The structure of an organization will affect the communication patterns, relationships and authority, so must be given due consideration and reviewed as an important part of any restructure or re-organization (Marquis and Huston 2009).

Link to Chapter 5 to discover more about the effect organizational structure has on communication.

Organization pyramid or hierarchical vertical structure

These are most common structures in healthcare Trusts. Employees are clear about the chain of command and authority. The hierarchical position in the organization is clear from looking at Figure 4.1. It is deliberate that Figure 4.1 does not include labels indicating job titles. It reflects the vertical structure of a large organization, with the Chief Executive at the top, with the second tier reflecting heads of departments. Equally, this structure can be applied to smaller, station-based teams. With station manager/team leader at the top, clinical managers/team leaders in tier 2 and paramedics in tier 3, there would be many more than the two boxes that are shown in Figure 4.1.

As you will realize through your additional reading, there are many organizational structures, which have been identified in various organizations and suit certain companies' business requirements. Walton (1997) uses the terminology of 'organization pyramid', where the hierarchy of job levels is clearly

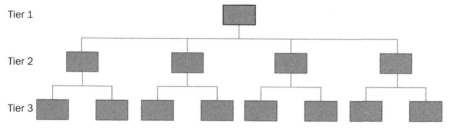

Figure 4.1 Representation of an organization pyramid or hierarchical vertical structure.

depicted, Barr and Dowding (2012) use the terminology 'hierarchical vertical structure'. Figure 4.1 only demonstrates a three-tier hierarchy, in reality, there would be many more levels, thus comprising a *tall* hierarchy. In times of financial constraint, this structure has the flexibility to be made quite *flat*. If this does occur, it is quite possible that a tier of senior managers may be removed, saving money and distributing their workload to others. This commonly happens in the NHS, in times of financial constraint and subsequent restructure.

Providing a visual representation is fine, but what cannot be demonstrated is the effect this type of structure has on communication and relationships, the human factors (this applies to any visual representation). Such tall structures have the potential to alienate employees, as they may feel they have no voice, as they are several rungs of the ladder away from anyone in authority. Communication is restricted and tends only to be 'top down', and this also discourages discussion and employee expression. Organizations with this structure need to consider the disadvantages and apply creative ways to overcome these potential harmful issues. Reduced staff morale is a real problem within healthcare settings and potentially affects the experience of the patient, and should be something that healthcare organizations consider seriously.

As Walton (1997) identifies, there is no indication of the inter-relationships of the second (and subsequent) tiers, or what would, in reality, be directorates. This structure encourages each director to look after their own domain, rather than creating a culture of collaboration and openness, indeed, there could even be competition for scarce resources. Figure 4.1 is too simplistic to explain how the decisions taken in one directorate would affect the whole organization. This level of complexity requires an in-depth examination of any one organization and all inter-relationships. But as Box 4.1 highlights, a change in any one area can substantially affect the organization and its efficiency or effectiveness.

Complex matrix structure of organizations

Barr and Dowding (2012) explain that the complex matrix structure can sometimes been seen within the NHS, when projects are being undertaken. This involves a cross-functional team, under several project managers. Smaller matrix teams may exist, with less of a hierarchy, such as community teams. In areas of the UK where paramedic community practitioners work with other allied health professionals, such as occupational therapists, physiotherapists, district nurses, this structure may be familiar, as part of the Ambulance Trust. In this situation, you would have a team leader and then team A, B, C, depending on the patient's location within the region (as shown in Figure 4.2). Characteristics of this structure are fewer levels of hierarchy, which should aid and improve communication. Marquis and Huston (2009) identify that decision-making in this structure can be slow, due to the necessity to liaise with others of the same managerial level. This

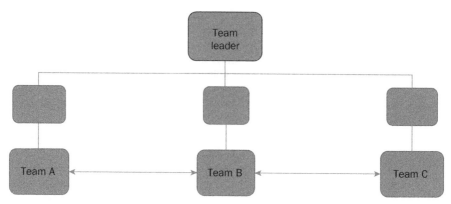

Figure 4.2 A complex matrix structure.

has the potential to cause frustration for employees. It also has the potential to be confusing for employees, when there is a dual command path, i.e. who do they approach, who is their manager?

It seems that this approach may become more prevalent, as the new Leadership model of 2013 recognizes the importance of working across organizational boundaries and improving integration between health and social care, primary and acute services (Storey and Holti 2013). This will require the leader in such a network context to understand others' perspectives, assess clients' needs in a holistic, rather than single agency manner, and build good relationships with other agencies. One of the nine dimensions of the Healthcare Leadership Model (2013) is entitled 'Connecting our service'. The four domains clearly articulate the importance being placed upon understanding your organization:

Essential	Recognizing how my area of work relates to other parts of the system
Proficient	Understanding the culture and politics across my organization
Strong	Adapting to different standards and approaches outside my organization
Exemplary	Working strategically across the system

The level of seniority/job role will dictate the level of competence expected of the staff member. To date, however, such organizational awareness has not been expressed in such detail.

Figure 4.2 implies some inter-communication between teams, this may or may not be the case, depending on the region served by the teams. However, there may be some staff movement between teams from time to time and communication where distances are less of a physical barrier.

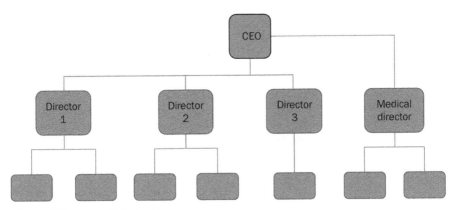

Figure 4.3   A parallel structure.

Parallel structure of organizations

Sullivan and Decker (2005) explain the parallel structure as being unique to healthcare settings. The development of the model is a result of the complex nature of senior healthcare managers and the authority of medical personnel. Historically, medical staff have resisted being *managed* by healthcare managers, this has led to some healthcare and Ambulance Trusts having parallel structures. This is probably less prevalent in Ambulance Trusts, but in some, a separate role of medical director exists within the management hierarchy. It is the way the individual holding this title liaises with the rest of the organization that is crucial. As seen in Figure 4.3, it has the danger of being isolated and being either too powerful or not effective within an organization, as there is the possibility of a lack of integration with other sections of the organization.

Reflection: points to consider

Examine the position of your medical director in your Trust, can you identify potential problems, or advantages?

It must be recognized that with the reforms of the NHS, this 'out on a limb' position of the medical director within the organizational structure is much less common now than it was in the 1990s. Many Trusts have successfully incorporated their medical colleagues under the organizational umbrella for the benefit of the work that the Trust is required to do and ultimately the benefit of patients. However, it is worth being aware of this historical perspective, as it may have shaped the structure of today's organization.

Organizational roles

Any organization will have a variety of roles at various levels within the hierarchy. All roles will involve working with other colleagues, to varying degrees. Some roles, generally the higher in the hierarchy, will be quite autonomous and in some cases isolating (depending on the post holder's personality and preference for working alone). Many roles in ambulance organizations involve working as part of a team, in many instances the teams are small, such as working as a crew. The increasing propensity for solo responders brings with it some potential issues, namely:

- safety concerns;

- risks associated with autonomous practice;

- opportunity to debrief;

- maintaining resilience in the long term.

This section of the chapter will specifically focus upon role adoption and the effect the organization has on the roles of teams and groups of people. The roles that individuals play within teams and groups of people and group dynamics are covered in Chapter 6.

Link to Chapter 6 for more information on group/team dynamics.

Role definition

In any organization there will be a wide variety of job roles, in order that the goals of the organization are met. These wider organizational goals are presented in the Trust's business plan, the mission statements, the Trust's vision. Job roles are usually defined by the production of a job description, where specific work and team roles are defined and specified. The fast pace of the changing workplace inevitably means that most job descriptions in the NHS are quite generic and lengthy, as exemplified by the paramedic profiles, which have been summarized for the purposes of this text. Usually only a few points are specific to varying job roles, usually related to professional experience, further education and skill level. For example, expected supervisory duties of paramedic (profile 2) vary depending on the 'presence of higher qualified healthcare professionals having a bearing on the degree of responsibility expected'. In the Specialist paramedic practitioner profile, the role taken is described as that of 'clinical leader, unless a more senior/ specialist professional was on scene'. In both examples, the paramedics clearly defer to colleagues who have a more appropriate set of skills for the patient's needs. More generally, expectations of role alter and change over time until a person leaves a role. Mullins (2005: 538) defines a *role* as 'an expected pattern of behaviour associated with members occupying a particular position within the structure of an organization'. Within the paramedic workforce of an organization, this is clearly visible within the chain of command, hierarchies of individual Trusts and the job titles of personnel.

Organizational citizenship behaviour

The concept of organizational citizenship behaviour (OCB) is one which readily applies to the ambulance service. Organ (1988: 57) explains that OCB focuses on the individual behaviour that is 'discretionary, not directly or explicitly recognized by the formal reward system, and that in the aggregate promotes the effective functioning of the organization'. For ambulance services, this can be explained by courtesy, smiling and other *customer-friendly* behaviours exhibited on a daily basis by Trust employees. The concept of OCB cannot be discussed without referring to the emotional labour of caring roles and the management of emotions. Obviously a healthcare organization wants and expects employees to manage emotions that are consistent with organizational and occupational expectations. Demonstration of empathy when caring for a patient is considered *emotional labour* (Larson and Yao 2005). This does not mean the employee feels this empathetic or emotionally positive internally, it may be nothing more than an outward demonstration of their professionalism. Internally, the employee may be emotionally troubled and be struggling to be at work and continue their usual duties. Storey and Holti (2013) believe such negative feelings and behaviours can become normalized within groups or the organization along with feelings of cynicism, anger, fear, anxiety, frustration and discontent. They see leaders as being key players in establishing more positive emotional sets, such as compassion, commitment, empathy and optimism. It is believed this can be achieved by employee engagement (King's Fund 2012; Alimo-Metcalf and Alban-Metcalf 2012). It will be a challenge for the paramedic profession to include paramedics who are lone workers and engage them in the dialogue proposed above. The leadership framework of 2013 will provide opportunities for involvement by the organization and staff should be encouraged to participate and be involved (Storey and Holti 2013).

Self-evaluation exercise

- Read the Leadership Academy's section on how to use the Leadership Framework to communicate the organization's vision. It can be accessed at: http://www.leadershipacademy.nhs.uk/wp-content/uploads/2012/11/NHSLeadership-LeadershipFramework-OrganizaationalToolkit-OrganizationalDevelopment.pdf.
- Do you recognize your Trust adopting some of these ideas?

The reality of employment

New registrants can feel quite unprepared for their first job, despite input from the higher education institute in terms of theory. The reality of being an employee (for some registrants for the first time) can be very different from what was expected or alluded to by the local employing NHS Ambulance Trust. Indeed, Kramer (1974) refers to *reality shock* and this still remains pertinent today. It is important for the new registrant and other staff to understand the importance of preceptorship in this transition period.

Link to Chapter 10 for more on preceptorship.

Many people talk about the *honeymoon* phase of new jobs. Schmalenburg and Kramer (1979) developed the four phases of role transition from student to practitioner further, also including *shock, recovery* and *resolution*. For many ambulance services the integration of paramedics who have been educated via the higher education (HE) route has been troublesome, in terms of challenging organizational culture and change of system, from vocational (IHCD) to HE (University). If it has been disconcerting for experienced paramedics, consider the challenge it has presented to newly registered paramedics who may sometimes be the most qualified person in an ambulance but the one lacking the most clinical experience, while trying to exert their leadership skills and do the best for the patient while battling strongly held beliefs and attitudes of colleagues. Kramer (1974) identified that this *reality shock* may see some clinical staff leave their jobs early in their careers. To avoid this, organizations and staff need to work together.

In very many cases experienced paramedics are a constant source of support and encouragement for new registrants. Organizations can support all concerned by providing both formal and informal mechanisms to assist staff in coming to terms with leading in the clinical area. Staff need to feel supported and valued by the organization. In a tall hierarchy, there is an inevitable distance between people in a management role and frontline clinical staff. There is also a potential for a lack of appreciation of the reality of the role of paramedic. With the hypothetical distance, a lack of communication between the hierarchies may occur. Support needs to be encouraged and prioritized for all staff, from the top of the organization. We have already mentioned the potential for sickness within ambulance staff, a support structure that is available to all and is effective is essential.

Link to Chapters 2 and 3 for more on leadership and Chapter 9 for more on conflict resolution, to explore what happens when teams do not get on.

Organizational culture

What is organizational culture? Unfortunately, there is no simple answer to this question. One aspect common to the literature is that it is a concept that is difficult to define, because of its multi-dimensional nature and lack of agreement between academics (Ott 1989; Jordan 1994; Mannion et al. 2008). Balogun and Hailey's (2004) definition of 'the way we do things around here' is simple, yet pertinent. Organizational culture can be a fairly abstract concept, I hope case study 4.2, and subsequent discussion, will prove illuminating and help to make the concept clearer. On discussion with undergraduate student paramedics, their first exposure to the *world of the paramedic* can be exciting, while conversely shocking at the same time.

Case study 4.2 is fictitious and has been developed after hearing many student paramedic accounts, where the reality of the world they have entered dawns on them. Students are encouraged to explore practice experiences and discuss them, in order that they are able to make some sense of their experience.

Case study 4.2

The student had attended a call to a home address, with their mentor (other crews also arrived). The patient was a young man, of a similar age to the student recalling the event. The young patient had suffered a sudden, traumatic death. The student could not believe the scene and was overwhelmed with emotion, while trying to act professionally and make sense of what could have led to the death of the young man.

The student paramedic recalled to the peer group, that the paramedics present were not really caring for the young man, but were looking around the room, commenting about the décor, the personal belongings that were in the room and making, what the student called, sick jokes.

The student ended their description of the event with the following sentence: 'I couldn't believe their responses, will I end up like that?'

There is an extensive discussion to be had around the factors that may have led to the paramedics' response, detailed in case study 4.2. In respect of culture, it is worth considering the following, rather wordy definition from Schein (1991: 111):

> Culture can be defined as a pattern of basic assumption, invented, discovered or developed by a given group, as it learns to cope with its

problems of external adaptation and internal integration, that has worked well enough to be considered valid and therefore to be taught to new members as the correct way to perceive, think and feel in relation to those problems.

Emergency services' coping mechanisms

It could be argued that coping strategies, both positive and negative, have been *invented, discovered and developed* by the paramedics in case study 4.2, in order to cope with this distressing event described by a student. It is recognized that this conversation was not in the presence of anyone, other than those *in the profession*, student or registered, so the student had experienced the first step *to internal integration*. I have no doubt that if the staff concerned had realized the effect these actions and words had on the student, they would have amended or diluted their reaction and response.

As emergency workers we often readily accept people into our world, but we must remember that for some time, it will be challenging, scary and potentially shocking for the newcomer. That is something that is easy to forget, as happened in case study 4.2, especially if the newcomer fits in quite quickly and conforms to cultural norms. It also needs to be recognized that this is one student's experience and the reactions of a few members of staff. It is well documented that coping strategies are not always positive or healthy, especially among emergency service workers (Boxer and Wild 1993; Gould and Greenberg 2008; Callaghan et al. 2000). The literature cites a mixture of strategies, such as poor diet, varied or poor sleeping patterns, reliance on alcohol, not accessing support networks and preferring to cope alone.

Surviving the organizational culture

During such reflective exercises students often explore instances that have shocked them and challenged their pre-student view of the ambulance service. This can often lead to a myriad of emotions, including emotional upset, anger and disbelief. This often leads to a closer examination of the issue via more discussion, reading and developing self-awareness. It is during such emotionally raw discussions that as academics we have valuable insight into the potential (or not) resilience of individual students. All higher education courses will (to varying degrees) address the issue of resilience. It is an extremely important area to consider and can be the difference between a student being successful and completing their course or dropping out. As an employee or a student, the tool of 360° feedback is useful to obtain an in-depth review of how others perceive you, and the CLCF self-assessment tool is useful for your continuing professional development.

Self-reflective exercises

- Follow the web link to the 360° feedback tool: http://www.leadershipacademy.nhs.uk/discover/leadership-framework-360-feedback-tool/.

- The CLCF self-assessment tool can be accessed via: http://www.leadershipacademy.nhs.uk/wp-content/uploads/2012/11/NHSLeadership-Framework-CLCFSelfAssessmentTool.pdf.

- The Healthcare Leadership Model can be accessed via: http://www.leadershipacademy.nhs.uk.

- For more on workplace well-being and self-help guides and worksheets, go to: www.businessballs.com/workplace-wellbeing.htm.

It appears that Ambulance Trusts have varying ways of approaching the support of employees. Sometimes it will not include student paramedics, as they are not employees, sometimes it will, but usually only when there is a structured debrief for an extreme incident. It does not have to be a large, multi-trauma incident that will bother a student, often it can be something that experienced paramedics will consider 'bread and butter' but has the potential to really make an impact on the student. In this situation, it is the skill of the paramedic educator (PEd) to assess the situation, the student's reactions and subsequent state of mind. Then they use their communication skills to encourage discussion and reflection. Obviously, passing relevant information onto the academic team is the key to continued support and follow-up, as time constraints or shift patterns will often prohibit the PEd's consistent supportive role. It must also be recognized by Ambulance Trusts and higher education institutions that PEds may require a forum for discussion and support, as some students will require a lot of emotional energy to be expended by the PEd.

Link to Chapter 10 for more on paramedic practice education and preceptorship.

The extreme and chaotic nature of the ambulance service can lead to what some people may describe as seemingly bizarre cultures. However, as the student in case study 4.2 discovered, exploring one experience can lead to interpretation, not necessarily understanding or acceptance of the organizational culture. Having provided a lengthy definition earlier, I would like to conclude this part of the chapter with a definition of organizational culture that is more succinct, 'culture is a lens through which an organization can be understood and interpreted' (Konteh et al. 2008: 205). What would an outsider see if they looked at your organization?

Self-reflective exercises

- Situate your position in the organization as a flow chart.
- How many roles or hierarchies are there in your management structure?
- What are the various directorates and departments in your Trust?
- Set these out as a flow chart. How do they link to each other?
- Think about the team of people who work with you, can you identify the role that individuals adopt within a team?
- What happens when you have two people who take on the same role?

Potential future developments

The complex nature of care in the twenty-first century requires a holistic approach from the NHS, in both hospital and community services. The future of ambulance services is likely to be consistently focused upon the care of the patient at home (as far as possible). This will require organizational changes in structure, in services offered and in liaison with other community professionals.

The new model of Leadership for the NHS (Storey and Holti 2013) suggests three innovations:

1. Service redesign that streamlines care and breaks down barriers between services and organizations.

2. Supporting patients and service users in managing their own care.

3. Changing ingrained patterns of behaviour in staff groups moving towards becoming more patient-centred.

If realized, these innovations will have a long-term effect on organizations, their structures and culture. For ambulance services, this may involve multi-professional teams working closely together and being employed by one organization, instead of several, as is generally the case now. Paramedics may be employed by GPs directly. This will, in turn, alter the existing culture of organizations and groups, providing new opportunities and challenges.

Conclusion

When the paramedic secures their first employment position within the NHS, they do not really consider how the employing organization may affect their motivation, sense of satisfaction with their role, feeling of being valued, and whether their views will be listened to and respected. As the paramedic's employment and career progresses, these issues become significantly more important. It is also crucial for any leader or manager to appreciate the importance of communication within the organization, the power of organizational culture, and its potential detrimental effects.

This chapter has introduced the influence that organizational history, structure and characteristics have on the culture of an organization. It has examined the above in respect of Ambulance Trusts as organizations within the NHS. Self-evaluation exercises, case studies and reflection points have been included to help the reader widen their perspective of the subject and help to facilitate understanding. Understanding the organization and all its various facets is important both for the employee and the employer, as it has the potential to ultimately affect patient care.

Chapter key points

- Organizations are shaped by their history. The present-day structures and cultures have developed over time.
- The theoretical characteristics of an organization can be seen within ambulance services, to varying degrees.
- Organizational structures will have an effect on employees, their motivation and ability to undertake their work in an efficient and effective way.
- The ambulance service, as with other parts of the NHS, has a unique culture.
- Ambulance services are unique as organizations and are distinct from other parts of the NHS, due to the nature and variety of the work, support networks and staff coping strategies.
- An examination of culture within organizations reveals both positive and negative aspects. This may affect how the employee works within the organization and how the organization is perceived by new recruits and students.
- Self-awareness and the development of resilience will help the reader cope with the demands of organizational life.

References and suggested reading

Alimo-Metcalf, B. and Alban-Metcalf, J. (2012) *Engaging Leadership: Creating Organisations that Maximise the Potential of their People*. London: CIPD.

Balogun, J. and Hailey, V.H. (2004) *Exploring Strategic Change*. London: Prentice Hall.

Barr, J. and Dowding, L. (2012) *Leadership in Health Care*, 2nd edn. London: Sage.

Bendall, C. (2012) Personal communication on the gender ratio within the paramedic profession, 19 March 2012.

Boxer, P.A. and Wild, D. (1993) Psychological distress and alcohol use among firefighters, *Scandinavian Journal of Environmental Health*,19(2): 121–5.

Business Dictionary.com (2013) Definition of an organisation. Available at: www.businessdictionary.com/definition/organization.html (accessed 18 August 2013).

Callaghan, P., Tak-Ying, S.A. and Wyatt, P.A. (2000) Factors related to stress and coping among Chinese nurses in Hong Kong, *Journal of Advanced Nursing*, 31(6): 1518–27.

Craggs, B. and Blaber, A.Y. (2008) Consideration of history, in A.Y. Blaber (ed.) *Foundations for Paramedic Practice: A Theoretical Perspective*. Maidenhead: McGraw-Hill/Open University Press.

Essex, B. and Benz-Scott, L. (2008) Chronic stress and associated coping strategies among volunteer EMS personnel, *Pre-hospital Emergency Care*, 12(1): 69–75.

Galbraith, J. (1977) *Organizational Design*. Reading, MA: Addison-Wesley.

Gould, M. and Greenberg, N. (2008) Patient characteristics and clinical activities at a British military department of community mental health, *The Psychiatrist*, 32: 99–102.

Jordan, A.T. (1994) Organizational culture: the anthropological approach, *National Association for the Practice of Anthropology Bulletin*, 14(1): 3–16.

King's Fund (2012) *Leadership and Engagement for Improvement in the NHS: Together We Can*. London: King's Fund.

Konteh, F.H., Mannion, R. and Davies, H.T.O. (2008) Clinical governance: views on culture and quality improvement, *Clinical Governance: An International Journal*, 13(3): 200–7.

Kramer, K. (1974) *Reality Shock: Why Nurses Leave Nursing*. Texas: Mosby.

Larson, E.B. and Yao, X. (2005) Clinical empathy as emotional labor in the patient–physician relationship, *Journal of the American Medical Association*, 293(9): 1100–6.

Lega, F. (2007) Organisational design for health integrated delivery systems: theory and practice, *Health Policy*, 81: 258–79.

Lindenburg, E. (2012) Patient and staff's perspectives on comfort touch in the care environment: implications for paramedic practice. Dissertation submission, as part of BSc (Hons) Paramedic Practice. University of Brighton. Unpublished.

Mannion, R., Davies, H., Konteh, F., Jung, T., Scott, T., Bower, P., Whalley, D., NcNally, R. and McMurray, R. (2008) *Measuring and Assessing Organisational Culture in the NHS*. Research Report. London: the National Co-ordinating Centre for the National Institute for Health Research Service Delivery and Organisation Programme (NCCSDO).

Marquis, B.L. and Huston, C. J. (2009) *Leadership Roles and Management Functions in Nursing*, 6th edn. Philadelphia, PA: Wolters Kluwer Health/Lippincott Williams & Wilkins.

Mildenhall, J. (2012) Occupational stress, paramedic informal coping strategies: a review of the literature, *Journal of Paramedic Practice*, 4(6): 318–28.

Mullins, L.J. (2005) *Management and Organisational Behaviour*, 7th edn. New York: Prentice Hall-Financial Times.

National Audit Office (2011) *Transforming NHS Ambulance Services*. Report by the Controller and Auditor General. HC 1086. Session 2010–2012. 10 June. London: Department of Health.

National Health Service Choices (2013) NHS choices website. London: NHS. Available at: http://www.nhs.uk/NHSEngland/thenhs/about/Pages/overview.aspx (accessed 18 September 2013).

Newton, A. (2012a) The ambulance service: the past, present and future, *Journal of Paramedic Practice*, 4(5): 303–5.

Newton, A. (2012b) The ambulance service: the past, present and future, *Journal of Paramedic Practice*, 4(6): 365–6.

NHS Leadership Academy (2013) *Healthcare Leadership Model: The Nine Dimensions of Leadership Behaviour.* Version 1.0. Leeds: NHS Leadership Academy. Available at: www.leadershipacademy.nhs.uk/leadershipmodel (accessed 26 November 2013).

Nursing and Midwifery Council (2012) *Statistics about Nurses and Midwives.* London: NMC. Available at: http://www.nmc-uk.org/About-us/Statistics/Statistics-about-nurses-and-midwives/ (accessed 1 February 2013).

Organ, D.N. (1988) *Organizational Citizenship Behavior: The Good Soldier Syndrome.* Lexington, MA: Lexington Books.

Ott, J.S. (1989) *The Organizational Culture Perspective.* Pacific Grove, CA: Brooks-Cole Publishing Company.

Parmelli, E., Flodgren, G., Schaafsma, M.E., Baillie, N., Beyer, F.R. and Eccles, M.P. (2011) *The Effectiveness of Strategies to Change Organisational Culture to Improve Healthcare Performance (Review).* The Cochrane Collaboration. New York: John Wiley and Sons.

Prati, G., Palestini, L. and Pietrantoni, L. (2009) Coping strategies and professional quality of life among emergency workers,. *The Australasian Journal of Disaster and Trauma Studies,* 1: 1–12.

Regehr, C. and Millar, D. (2007) Situation critical: low control, and low support in paramedic organisations, *Traumatology,* 13(49): 49–58.

Richardson, R. (1974) *Larrey: Surgeon to Napoleon's Imperial Guard.* London: Quiller Press.

Savage, J. (2000) The culture of 'culture' in National Health Service policy implementation, *Nursing Inquiry,* 7: 230–8.

Schein, E.H. (1991) *Organisational Culture and Leadership.* San Francisco: Jossey-Bass.

Schmalenburg, C. and Kramer, M. (1979) *Coping with Reality Shock.* Amherst, MA: Nursing Resources.

Storey, J. and Holti, R. (2013) *Towards a New Model of Leadership for the NHS.* The Open University Business School for the NHS Leadership Academy. Available at: http://www.leadershipaceademy.nhs.uk (accessed 13 August 2013).

Sullivan, E.J. and Decker, P.J. (2005) *Effective Leadership and Management in Nursing,* 6th edn. Harlow: Pearson Education Limited.

Suserud, B.O. (2005) Culture and care in the Swedish ambulance services, *Emergency Nurse,* 13(8): 30–6.

Walton, M. (1997) *Management and Managing,* 2nd edn. Cheltenham: Stanley Thornes.

PART 2
The skills of leadership

5 Communication
Its impact on leadership
Paul Street

In this chapter

- Introduction
- Leadership and communication
- Communication theory relevant to paramedics in NHS ambulance services
- Verbal techniques
- Non-verbal behaviours
- Active listening
- Messages
- The effect of encoding and decoding
- Context of communication
- Leadership style and communication
- Power and position
- Organizational communication and leadership
- Communication systems
- Written communication
- Radio or telephone communication
- Electronic and computer-assisted communication
- Conclusion
- Chapter key points
- References and suggested reading
- Useful website

Introduction

Communication and leadership are inextricably linked and completely co-dependent (Barr and Dowding 2012; Kotter 2012); further, how leaders communicate can have a direct effect on the quality of clinical care, on service development and on how a team works together (World Health Organisation 2009) and the speed of actions that follow communication (Forsyth 2012).

Post the Francis Report (2013) and the government's response in *Patients First and Foremost* (Department of Health 2013), it is evident that good leaders should have a pivotal role in promoting good quality care ensuring that Health Service organizations are safe and deliver individualized care, with good communication and leadership being fundamental to this. It is difficult to think of any situation in which ambulance clinicians are involved that does not include communication and some sort of leadership, from providing care to organizational development. Therefore, good leaders communicate and promote high quality care. So ambulance clinicians need to have both effective communication skills alongside the appropriate facilities to communicate in order to lead clinical practice, the ambulance service and the paramedic profession (Gregory and Ward 2010; HCPC 2012).

Throughout the many excellent interactions that occur daily within the ambulance service, the potential for misunderstanding and miscommunication in all clinical and leadership situations remains. This is particularly the case, if consideration is not given to how and what needs to be communicated and the effect that any particular context will have on the process and outcome of communication (Barr and Dowding 2012). In total, the NHS receives over 3000 written complaints a week, many of which are to do with communication (Health & Social Care Information Centre 2012). Also the Francis Report has highlighted the vital role communication has for patients and healthcare organizations alike, in either promoting or inhibiting the quality of care and the effectiveness of organizational leadership (The Stationery Office 2013). Thus, communication and leadership are important for all paramedics, irrespective of their level within service (Martin and Swinburn 2012).

Leadership and communication

Traditionally leaders have been categorized by the traits or charisma they exhibit or by the appointed position they hold, with staff in subordinate positions following their leadership (Cole and Kelly 2011). However, the NHS Leadership Academy (2013) Healthcare Leadership Model has moved beyond these traditional perspective and promotes a shared view of leadership, in which all staff have some leadership qualities and behaviours that contribute to leadership in some way, and in this system, communication is critical. Communication is not just about giving instructions, it is a mechanism for creating vision, giving direction and enhancing motivation too (Barr and Dowding 2012). There are hierarchical elements in leadership roles in the ambulance service, for example, Senior paramedic, Specialist paramedic, Advanced paramedic, and Consultant paramedic among other managerial positions, as detailed in the paramedic profiles at the beginning of this book. These positions deliver a leadership function by providing specialist knowledge, skill or service direction and are guided by the expectations and patterns of behaviour for those roles, but communication is fundamental to all of them (Barr and Dowding 2012; HCPC 2012; Martin and Swinburn 2012). If paramedics at all levels had both the technical and non-technical skills (see Box 5.1), they would have significant leadership potential in terms of role modelling professional behaviours and facilitating the ethos of professional practice, enhancing quality and developing the service (Taylor and Armitage 2012). For example, one paramedic may demonstrate leadership qualities when assessing a patient in their home, while another may lead a team in a complex road traffic incident, while another leads a service development, or acts as a role model for a student paramedic.

Box 5.1   Non-technical skills attributed to communication

- Communication
- Situational awareness
- Decision-making
- Teamwork
- Managing stress

Source: Taylor and Armitage (2012).

Link to Chapters 1 and 3 for more discussion on the NHS Leadership Framework.

Communication theory relevant to paramedics in NHS ambulance services

The ambulance service is a complex organization that is dependent on communication at all levels to ensure that calls are received, practitioners are dispatched, patients are assessed, and services led, planned and provided (Gregory and Ward 2010). Furthermore, the World Health Organisation (2009) argues that communication and leadership are crucial elements of patient safety.

At the most fundamental level, communication is the transfer of information from one person or place to another (Barr and Dowding 2012). The most rudimentary model of interpersonal communication proposes that a sender sends a message that is received by a receiver (Ellis 2003). The sender will have a thought to communicate, will formulate that into a message and then send it to the receiver, using verbal and non-verbal means of communication. The receiver will then respond and communicate feedback to the initial sender (see Figure 5.1).

However, there are a myriad of interpersonal issues that influence how the message has been formulated (*encoded*) by the sender and understood

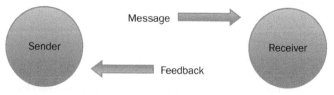

Figure 5.1   Fundamental model of communication.

(*decoded*) by the receiver as seen in Figure 5.1. It is the interrelationship between encoding and decoding that can result in misunderstanding of the initial message and the response. The principles of both models apply in any situation where communication occurs, including leadership at clinical or strategic levels (WHO 2009; NHS Leadership Academy 2011).

Verbal techniques

All good leaders use a mixture of verbal and non-verbal communication skills to maximize the potential for communicating a message, whether that is leading a clinical situation or a service development (Barr and Dowding 2012). Verbal communication is often thought to be the primary means of communication (Hogg and Vaughan 2010) and in most healthcare situations spoken verbal communication figures very highly as a means of communication, though Mehrabian (1981) suggests that only 7% of the meaning of any message, when communicating emotions, is attributed to the actual words used. Verbal communication has two main elements: the words themselves and then the modulation of the way the words are spoken, i.e. the paralinguistic features such as tone, pitch and intonation (see Table 5.1).

To clearly communicate in any situation, the paramedic needs to consider what they need to say and how they should say it, to maximize the effectiveness of that communication, particularly if they are leading a situation in some way. The type of language used in any situation is the conscious decision of the person communicating, even if the subsequent meaning and interpretation of those words are not (Hogg and Vaughan 2010). In most situations, the clearer the language used, the easier the communication (Forsyth 2012). Therefore, when dealing with patients, all paramedics should use terms that the patient and their families can understand and avoid the use of technical terms, jargon and abbreviations (HCPC 2012). This would have the advantage that everyone in a situation, other paramedics, emergency services and patients and their family, will potentially understand the meaning of any communication. In this way clear instructions can be given

Table 5.1 Features of communication and non-technical leadership skills underpinned by communication

Paralinguistic features	Non-verbal features
Volume	Eye contact
Rhythm	Facial expression
Pitch	Gestures
Pace	Posture
Intonation	Position
Tone	Proximity
Repetition	Touch
	Smell
	Appearance
	Uniform

and clinical leadership demonstrated, minimizing the potential for misunderstanding. In the case of time-critical situations, the use of abbreviations and medical terms can speed up communication (Fellows and Woolcock 2009), though there is the potential risk if the patient is conscious that they will feel excluded and their anxiety will increase, because they do not understand what is happening to them. In such situations, when appropriate, it would be advisable to regularly include the patient and their family in the conversation, keeping them up-to-date with what is happening. But here the practitioner has to decide what is in the patient's best interest, being included or prioritizing care. Verbal communication is important in the paramedic team, as case study 5.1 highlights.

Case study 5.1

Student paramedics are consistently asked to evaluate their experience in practice and are encouraged to provide ideas on how to improve their mentor–student relationship.

State one thing your mentor could change that would affect your practice experience.

This is the question posed to all student paramedics annually and their answers consistently reflect the practice environment, specifically the vehicle and the problems it poses for students in respect of paralinguistic and non-verbal communication.

Many students comment that their mentor and colleagues travel to all calls in the front of the vehicle, with the student in the rear of the vehicle. This significantly affects the student paramedic's ability to hear all the verbal communication, via the radio and between colleagues. The student very often misses vital pieces of information relating to the patient and circumstances of the call and certainly is not in a position to hear the subtleties of paralinguistic features, such as tone and intonation. Early in the student–mentor relationship the student often does not have the confidence to ask colleagues to repeat what they have said, so the student often goes to a call, unprepared or missing vital information. In one student example, the word 'hanging' was not heard, so the student entered the premises mentally unprepared for the situation they found themselves in.

In order for the student paramedic to give their best, they need to hear all the information that the crew have available to them. They also need to be party to the crew's plan once they arrive and feel prepared for the situation and be part of the team, and communication is vital to all of these aspects of care. All students recognize they are not the most important part of the team. As one student said: 'Travelling in the rear of the vehicle all the time may seem a small thing, but it affects what I can hear, how I prepare myself, my learning and feeling outside of the team. It would be nice if we could alternate who sat in the back of the vehicle.'

Is this something for mentors to be aware of?

Link to Chapter 3 for more information about clinical leadership.

Paralinguistic features

Paralinguistic features are an integral part of verbal communication and are used to shape the sound and meaning of the language. It is evident that speaking clearly and precisely can significantly help reduce the risk of ambiguity, thus decreasing the risk of misunderstanding (Taylor 2012) and this should form the basis of all spoken communication and leadership situations. In addition to the vocal clarity, how words are spoken is also important. Changes in intonation, tone, pitch and volume can be used to communicate a range of meanings, for example, compassion, frustration or a sense of urgency. In terms of leadership, these changes should demonstrate positive communication attributes rather than negative ones and affirm the meaning of the words rather than layering other meanings onto the words (Gregory and Ward 2010). Even if you are giving bad news to a patient or to a colleague, the intonation should be an empathetic one, concurrent with the news (Fellows and Woolcock 2009). However, some of the changes in tone and intonation, for example, occur as a result of an emotional response to a situation, while in other situations they are under the direct control of the sender (Hogg and Vaughan 2010). Nevertheless, in all situations it is feasible to have some element of control over the paralinguistic features. For example, in stressful situations, people tend to talk louder and faster than normal. Here it would be possible for you to consciously lower your volume and slow the pace at which you talk, therefore sounding calmer than you might be. However, the volume used to send a message needs to be appropriate to the situation, a noisy accident scene would require a higher volume than when in a meeting room setting, too loud and the person may think you are shouting at them, too soft and they may not hear you at all. So an inappropriate volume level could adversely affect the interpretation of the message. Closely linked to volume is pitch, usually the louder the volume, the higher the pitch of voice. If these two elements are then linked to a fast pace of speaking, these could then paralinguistically communicate a sense of urgency, panic or frustration (Hogg and Vaughan 2010). Thus, the possible consequences for ambulance practitioners using a raised volume, pitch and pace are that the people receiving the message may perceive the situation as serious, or that they are being told off or reprimanded in some way. These changes may be, in part, due to alterations in the practitioner's anxiety levels during any patient interaction, particularly if it is a stressful one. Additionally, the more the practitioner feels under pressure, the more these features may appear in the voice. Hence, controlling the voice and having a calm paced rhythm and tone in their voice at an appropriate volume may then communicate confidence (Bledsoe *et al.* 2010) particularly in complex situations. For example, in time-critical situations in a patient's home or in the call centre where the dispatcher is dealing with a very anxious person over the phone who needs reassurance while undertaking any instructions given by the dispatcher, such as when and how to do cardiac compressions. Here, if the dispatcher sounds calm and confident, then it is more likely that the caller will respond positively to this and follow the instructions given or, at least, prevent their anxiety from increasing further.

Reflection: points to consider

Think about occasions when familiar colleagues have raised their voice in clinical situations:

• Which of these situations would you classify as stressful?

• Was your colleague in a leadership role in these clinical situations?

• Just because you did not find the situation stressful, put yourself in your colleague's position, does this change your view?

Link to Chapter 6 to read more about teamworking.

Self-evaluation exercise

Complete Section 1 of the NHS Leadership Academy's self-assessment activity 'Demonstrating personal qualities'. This may provide you with more self-awareness and insight into areas of your personality that are strong or may require development. This can be accessed at: http://www. leadershipacademy.nhs.uk/wp-content/uploads/2012/11/NHSLeadership-Framework-LeadershipFrameworkSelfAssessmentTool.pdf.

Non-verbal behaviours

Non-verbal communication, in a similar way to the paralinguistic features of verbal communication, can enhance, supplement, contradict or replace the meaning of the verbal message being sent (Ellis 2003), particularly as 55 per cent of the meaning of any interaction is conveyed by non-verbal behaviours (Mehrabian 1981). Many non-verbal behaviours are unconscious manifestations of thoughts and feelings and therefore uncontrollable (Hartley 1999). Nevertheless, many non-verbal behaviours can be consciously controlled and used to help reinforce verbal messages or portray a particular impression, i.e. wanting to appear confident when nervous. This would be important in a clinical leadership situation when the patient and relatives may be scared, when any paramedic would need to appear confident, knowledgeable and skilful, because evident nervousness on behalf of the paramedic could show in their non-verbal and vocal cues (Fellows and

Woolcock 2009) and thus limit their clinical leadership potential. Similarly, if a senior paramedic was making a presentation at an international conference and they felt nervous, they could slow their speech, and stand in a confident position to appear more confident than they are. However, the danger here is that people may over-compensate and appear over-confident when they are really just nervous. So the key is self-awareness and getting a subtle balance of controlling non-verbal cues right.

Reflection: points to consider

- Have you ever mentored a student paramedic who appeared over-confident, but had little or no knowledge or skill they could apply to the situation?
- Do you think they could have just been very nervous, but not self-aware enough to obtain the right balance of non-verbal cues?
- Consider how you appear to others when you are nervous.

In conjunction with eye contact, the face is one of the most expressive parts of a human body (Borg 2008) and feelings like anger, frustration and disapproval are quite often easy to identify through facial expressions, by both patients and colleagues (Bickley and Szilagi 2007). Further, the position or angle of the head can also communicate meaning (Hartley 1999). Tilting the head forward combined with looking over the top of a pair of glasses can be seen as intimidating, while inclining the head to one side slightly can be perceived as a sign of interest. The latter, in combination with a smile, is way that ambulance clinicians can show they are interested in their patients and the people they lead (Bledsoe *et al.* 2010). Therefore, leaders in all situations need to consider what they are commutating facially, along with their other non-verbal and verbal messages, to ensure they are all consistent, to avoid misunderstanding.

Active listening

As a leader, it would be vital for you to ensure that the people you communicate with also feel that you are listening to them. If paramedics do not listen carefully, they may make ill-informed judgements (Fellows and Woolcock 2009), whether that is about patient care or other elements of their role, thus demonstrating poor leadership qualities (WHO 2009). It is generally accepted that, if possible, when talking to patients, ambulance clinicians should use an open posture, i.e. not having your arms or legs crossed, because often standing with your arms crossed in front of a patient or relative can be seen as confrontational and uncaring (Bledsoe *et al.* 2010). Both posture and gestures can have a positive effect on establishing and maintaining good communication, especially if used in combination with eye contact. If these are used appropriately, they can suggest you are concerned for the patient and are willing to listen to them, but if used unwisely, like prolonged or minimal eye contact, they can also alienate a patient, relative or colleague too because they can suggest you could be uncaring and unwilling to listen (Fellows and Woolcock 2009).

Reflection: points to consider

- As a mentor, do you give your student paramedic feedback on their posture and gestures after a call to a patient? Many student paramedics will not be used to starting a conversation with a stranger, they may benefit from some constructive feedback.
- In a non-emergency situation, do you actively listen, or are you busy *doing things* to a patient?
- How might this be perceived by the patient and significant others?

Self-evaluation exercise

Access Section 2 'Working with others' of the NHS Leadership Academy's self-assessment activity. This includes communication within the exercise. It can be accessed at: http://www.leadershipacademy.nhs.uk/wp-content/uploads/2012/11/NHSLeadership-Framework-Leadership-FrameworkSelfAssessmentTool.pdf.

Messages

Communication is most effective when it is kept clear and simple (Gregory and Ward 2010), but the challenge with this is that it takes time, thought and craft to construct meaningful clear messages (Kotter 2012) because communication is only truly effective when the receiver understands the precise meaning of the message the sender intended (Fellows and Woolcock 2012). If you have to say 'What I meant was', there has been an issue with either the clarity of the message or the interpretation of your original message (Forsyth 2012). Direct messages are those that have a single meaning and there are no inconsistencies between the literal meanings of the words, the paralinguistic features applied to the words and the non-verbal behaviours. Direct messages are the type that should be used in all leadership and clinical situations, ensuring the potential for miscommunication and misunderstanding is minimized (Kotter 2012).

When a consultant paramedic is preparing a presentation for the Trust board about a service development or the results from an audit, for example, they would have the time in advance to prepare what they want to say, to decide which paralinguistic features to use and consider what language they need to use with the Trust board and whether to reinforce their verbal message with written text and images in a PowerPoint presentation and written report. Such preparation would allow them to clearly prepare and craft their message, to be clear, concise and unambiguous. However, the paramedic would also need to consider the effect that the situation has on their communication abilities and control any undesirable elements such as appearing nervous, or speaking too quickly, for example. However, many leadership situations are not planned and occur in practice situations, where a high level of preparation of the message is not possible, as in case study 5.2. Here the paramedic needs to rely on their interpersonal and clinical skills to listen, assess and respond to the situation to lead it to a positive conclusion. Forsyth (2012) argues that the clarity of the message can significantly affect what occurs next. If the message is clearly articulated and accurately understood, it could speed up actions and improve efficacy, this would be particularly important when leading in a clinical situation where actions may be time-critical, for example, when a paramedic is dealing with a cardiac arrest situation in someone's home or when a call handler is having to give instructions to a person whose partner is giving birth. Here clear direct messages are the most effective. However, due to a variety of influences, messages may not be this clear, for example, stress, lack of understanding, all of which are demonstrated in case study 5.2.

Case study 5.2

During his first week with his mentor, David, a first year student paramedic, attended a call to a critically injured patient. David's mentor is a registered paramedic, the other member of the crew is a non-registered clinician. On their arrival, the non-registered clinician was directed by the paramedic, to apply pressure to an area of bleeding.

David is asked by his mentor 'to fetch the orange bag' from the vehicle. Sensing the gravity of the situation, David runs to the vehicle. He has sensed the urgency and picked up on the tone of his mentor's voice. David picks up the first orange bag that he finds. He returns to the patient and is shouted at by his mentor, 'Not that one, the other one, you idiot!'

- Think about this situation. Who is at fault?
- Why was there a miscommunication?
- What could have the mentor said to make his instruction clearer?
- Could David have done anything differently?

Messages with multiple meanings are common in daily communication, not only because all messages are open to a range of influences that can layer different meanings into one message, but because of the deliberate intentions of the both sender and receiver, for example, the use of sarcasm and humour. Humour used wisely could be an effective communicative tool to calm a situation or put a point across in a memorable way, so may have a place in some leadership situations, but using it runs the risk of alienating people if they do not understand the humour (Astedt-Kurki and Isola 2001). Sarcasm, however, should not be knowingly used in any leadership situations, as it essentially devalues the person you are talking to and therefore, limits positive leadership. However, sometimes when under pressure, some ambulance clinicians may be tempted to use it if they feel the caller or patient is using the service unnecessarily, or a colleague is being negative about a service development.

Reflection: points to consider

Think about a practice situation where communication suffered and affected the outcome for the patient. Would have changing the way the messages were delivered prevented the situation worsening?

The effect of encoding and decoding

The construction and interpretation of messages is a complex process and is influenced by both human factors and social influences like gender, personality, class, culture, education values and belief systems, all of which are influenced through an individual's primary, secondary and professional socialization (Hogg and Vaughan 2010; Blaber 2012; Taylor 2012). These factors affect the way the sender encodes a message and the receiver decodes it, and are apparent in the words, speech patterns, intonation, body language and behaviours used to send a message to give it the required meaning as perceived by the sender (Hartley 1999). It is the difference between these influences that is the most likely cause of misunderstanding, poor communication or limited leadership. Even if the paramedic message was clear, in terms of their values and beliefs, it may not be in terms that the receiver understands, as with case study 5.2. So when the message is decoded, in light of the receiver's own social factors, a misunderstanding may occur and they then send a seemingly inappropriate response back to the sender. This could occur when actually both messages could have been clear and direct, so the potential for a mismatch in understanding based on social influences is immense (Hogg and Vaughan 2010). If a paramedic is leading a situation and they treat every patient, person or colleague as an individual, and do not make value-based judgements, based on what is seen, said or assumed in a situation, the risk of miscommunication is reduced. So the paramedic is required to use good communication and listening skills to establish what is acceptable to do, say and ask in any situation. Furthermore, how an individual perceives themselves can also influence the way they encode and decode messages. If they perceive themselves as being vulnerable or confident, this may then influence how they perceive the situation and whether they feel in control or not. Thus self-perception can influence how people behave and respond to communication in any given situation (Taylor 2012).

Context of communication

The context in which communication and leadership occur will also influence the effect it has on the situation (see Box 5.2) and the perceived levels of leadership (Kotter 2012). Initially the physical environment will either promote or inhibit leadership clinically or organizationally, because of the resources and hazards within that situation. Demonstrating clinical leadership in a patient's home or over the telephone has different pressures and influences than those in a meeting with colleagues. Paramedics in the home or at a scene would have to take control and modify the physical environment more often than call handlers, because the call centre is designed for its function, while the home is not designed as a healthcare facility.

Box 5.2   Examples of some situational factors that could affect communication and leadership

- Personal and team cultures
- One to one interaction
- Somatic differences
- Different perceptions of a situation
- Selection perception of a situation
- Time pressures and deadlines
- Physical environment (stairs, furniture, animals, etc.)
- Psychological elements
- Stress
- Urgency
- Complexity
- Degree of threat, physical or psychological
- Type of environment
- Factors within that environment
- Team dynamics
- Relationships
- Status, hierarchies, power, position
- Different communication styles and abilities
- Cultural differences (personal, professional and organizational)
- Workload

- Fatigue
- Crisis situations
- Distractions (noise, people, other activities)
- Conflict
- Lack of privacy or personal space
- Technology
- Computer systems (PowerPoint, AMPDS)
- Radio equipment/poor reception or transmission
- Global positioning systems
- Tracking systems

Furthermore, the psychological elements will also affect communication (Fellows and Woolcock 2009). Both the call handlers and paramedics in the home would be influenced by the degree of urgency in the situation, the reactions of the patient and their family. However, the call handler will have to deal with one person via the telephone over a prolonged period of time until the paramedic arrives, while the crew will potentially have more than one anxious person and any other hazards at the scene. Therefore, both clinicians will need clear and unambiguous communication, often in tandem with assertive leadership, to allow the paramedic to assess and guide the people within that situation.

Potentially there are situations that escalate, for example, if a relative has been on the telephone with the call handler for some while, they would have gained large amounts of information about the situation. When the paramedic arrives and asks 'What has happened?' the relative could then get angry because they are going to have to repeat the information already given to the call handler. This could then lead to a more complex situation requiring good communication and leadership skills to defuse it. A consultant paramedic in a clinical governance meeting will face pressures, even though they only have an indirect influence on care at this point. The consultant paramedic will have an influence on colleagues' feelings and control over their response to the other people in the meeting. Their skill at communicating their report or findings may result in resistance to or approval of their plans.

Common to all of these situations is the issue of selective attention (Barr and Dowding 2012). This occurs when people only listen to the part of the message they want to hear, rather than the message in full. This is in addition to any information they do not hear due to factors in the physical and psychological environment. Hence, Kotter (2012) argues that good leaders use multiple methods to disseminate and gain information to minimize this effect, which may be easier in organizational leadership situations, than situations in a patient's home.

Reflection: points to consider

Think about any situation where you have not heard all of the message, this does not have to be in a work situation.

- Examine why you did not hear all of the message, were there external factors, such as environmental noise, for example, or did you think you had heard all of the message and *switched off*?
- What were the consequences?

Link to Chapter 3 for more detail on clinical leadership in the NHS and Chapter 8 for information about leading change.

Leadership style and communication

Leadership style can also influence the degree and type of communication (Barr and Dowding 2012). If the paramedic has an autocratic style of leadership, their communication may be very directive and they would very much take control of the situation and the people in it. They may ask direct questions to gain the key information they require, to assess the situation and identify what needs to be done, by whom, at what time, but may not facilitate much discussion. This, in some situations, would be highly effective leadership when taking control and managing the people are imperative, for example, in time-critical situations. People would probably be clear in terms of what they need to do, but they may not feel that they can contribute anything else apart from what they are asked to do. For individual situations, this would be effective. But if used in the long term, this could start to alienate work colleagues, as their contribution would be limited or the team would be disempowered because their contributions are not wanted or valued. Therefore, the leader does not have a team that can be independent when the leader is not there.

An alternative form of leadership would be a democratic one (Barr and Dowding 2012), where the leader leads by example, encouraging the people in the situation to contribute to the management and resolution of it. Here the communication skills require focus on collecting information by asking questions and active listening, appearing approachable, yet still being assertive enough to guide the situation. It would be more likely that the paramedic would appear more compassionate and engender a greater therapeutic or team working relationship. However, there is room for both these styles and that would depend on the context of the situation in which leadership is required. The higher the degree of urgency, the higher the need for a greater degree of authoritative leadership style. The art would be knowing when to use either of these styles depending on the situation. These autocratic and democratic elements of leadership are also apparent when leading in other situations such as meetings or working groups and the same principles apply.

> **Link to Chapter 6 for discussion on group dynamics and teamworking.**

Power and position

Without doubt, every paramedic, by the virtue of their education, role, position and uniform, carries a degree of power (Cole and Kelly 2011). How paramedics communicate can reduce, or increase, the inherent level of power they have, certainly in a clinical leadership situation (Gregory and Ward 2010). The degree of power changes depending on the situation they find themselves in, for example, in a meeting with a range of paramedics, a newly qualified clinician may feel they have less power than a Consultant paramedic. If the meeting was about implementing the results of an audit, then the Senior paramedic could take the autocratic approach saying: 'This is what we found and this is what we are going to do.' Here the message may be very clear, in terms of the findings, but also in terms of limiting the room for discussion and negotiation. However, for many patients, any ambulance consists of a paramedic and by virtue of that, they give an inherent power base to the clinician, because the patient often will not have the level of knowledge and skill that the paramedic does.

Reflection: points to consider

- Have you ever, in any non-urgent patient interaction, felt the patient is asking too many questions?
- Explore why you may have thought this.
- Was your feeling appropriate or, on reflection, were you unconsciously exploiting your position of power and adopting an 'I know best, so why are you asking me all these questions?' attitude, without knowingly doing so?

Organizational communication and leadership

A key element of leadership is evident in how the organization works and communicates (Barr and Dowding 2012) as it provides the means for all information, strategies, policies, goals and practices to be disseminated, discussed and implemented (Cole and Kelly 2011). Kotter (2012) suggests that organizations do not communicate enough to ensure that key messages are disseminated through an organization consistently, whether that is essentially a *top-down* or *bottom-up* approach to communication and leadership.

A top-down approach suggests that the organization will provide the employees with the information they need, while a bottom-up approach suggests that employees contribute to the process of communication and leadership by providing feedback about the information they are provided. Because the ambulance service is a complex organization, with a degree of hierarchy, it is inevitable that there are elements *of top-down* communication. However, Barr and Dowding (2012) suggest that organizations that facilitate both upward and downward communication often have the strongest leaders, because of the two-way communication. Moreover, Cole and Kelly (2011) argue, to maximize organizational communication, leaders should use the language of the person they are talking to, so if that is a patient, use lay terms, if it is a consultant in Emergency Care, use medical terminology. If it is a fellow paramedic, use medical terminology and localized ambulance service terms. This has the advantage of speeding up conversations, ensuring that the potential for clear communication is maximized and the resultant actions from that conversation are successful (Forsyth 2012), providing that no assumptions about the level of knowledge and understanding have been made. Therefore, the leader is required to actively listen to the person to whom they are talking and check that the message they are sending is the one they intend to send. So techniques like summarizing, clarifying and questioning are important communication and leadership strategies.

> **Link to Chapter 4 for more discussion about the organization and organizational culture.**

Communication systems

There are a range of tools that could help aid communication, some are based on information technology (IT), others could form part of documentation or be included in the principles of assessment (see Box 5.3), but they all contribute to the chain of communication, whether that is in leadership or clinical situations. Assessment tools like SBAR allow for the collection and transfer of focused information, while SOLER presents a framework for managing non-verbal behaviours, both of which contribute to the clarity of communication and therefore have a positive contribution to clinical leadership and patient safety (Gregory and Ward 2010).

Box 5.3   Tools to aid communication

- SBAR (Situation, Background, Assessment, Recommendation)
- SOLER (Squarely face the person, Open posture, Lean forward, Eye contact, Relax)
- SOAP (Subjective data, Objective data, Assessment Data, Plan of patient management)
- ASHICE (Age, Sex, History, Injures, Condition, Estimated time of arrival).

Reflection: points to consider

- Which of the tools in Box 5.3 are you familiar with?
- Examine the others, could they add anything extra to your handover technique?
- Would adding extra elements from other tools contribute to patient safety?

The NHS Institute for Innovation and Improvement (2008) has provided a template for using SBAR within clinical practice (see Table 5.2). In this framework, the situation section deals with basic information like names, places and the type of incident. This allows you to give a quick and accurate introduction. This leads you on to give a more detailed background about the patient and what has happened. Within the assessment section you deal with how you have assessed the patient and the situation and what conclusions you have reached. Finally, you would need to communicate what you recommend should happen now. This kind of tool would clearly help communication in terms of clinical leadership demonstrated by all levels of paramedic, because the communication is potentially clear and accurate. This approach, however, could easily be used in all formal situations when communication and leadership are required. If a Consultant paramedic was outlining a service development to a group of paramedics, they could easily structure their briefing around giving an overview of the situation in terms of the service development, what the background to it was and what has led up to the need for the development. Then discuss how the situation was assessed and what decisions were made. Then recommend a way forward, in terms of what needs to be done now.

Written communication

Written communication provides a valuable way of initiating or reinforcing messages in leadership situations. Barr and Dowding (2012) suggests that in terms of communicating key leadership messages using a mixed method of verbal, written and visual methods would help people in the organization take in those messages more effectively than using just one method. This maximizes the exposure of that message, but can also *link into* different individuals' learning and thinking styles. In most clinical situations a paramedic would be recording their assessment and actions either manually or electronically to ensure that all key information is documented and this provides a record of the care, aiding communication between paramedics and other healthcare providers, as well as a base for quality improvement, audit or research (Gregory and Ward 2010). Whatever the means of recording care, it would need to be clear, concise and accurate. This may in part be facilitated by the type of documentation, for example, in the Patient Report

Table 5.2 SBAR in a clinical and leadership situation

SBAR in a clinical leadership situation: Patient assessment	SBAR applied to a leadership situation: Giving feedback on an audit
(S) Situation • Identify yourself. • Identify the patient by name. • Give the specific details about the situation e.g. patient involved in a road traffic collision. • Give any details of initial vital signs, oxygen given, level of consciousness, etc. • Describe your concerns.	**(S) Situation** • Identify yourself. • Identify others involved. • Give the specific details about the situation. • Give any details of initial assessment of the situation and need for the audit. • Describe your concerns.
(B) Background • Give the patient's reason for admission. • Explain significant medical history. • Current medication and allergies. • Procedures you have undertaken. • Medications given by you and those normally taken by the patient. • Treatments/procedures you have undertaken.	**(B) Background** • Give the details of the situation, prior to the audit. • Outline the procedures and strategies you have undertaken to resolve the initial issues. • Outline how the audit was undertaken.
(A) Assessment • Vital signs. • Contraction pattern. • Clinical impression and concerns.	**(A) Assessment** • Outline the findings of the audit. • Outline if the strategies have resolved the issues. • Outline any emerging issues/ unresolved issues. • Outline your impression, conclusion and concerns.
(R) Recommendations • Explain what you think the patient needs now. • Make suggestions. • Clarify expectations.	**(R) Recommendations** • Explain what you think needs to be done now. • Make suggestions. • Clarify expectations.

Source: NHS Institute for Innovation and Improvement (2008) template for SBAR.

Form (PRF) used in many ambulance services. This requires minimal narrative, but a comprehensive check box system of recording care. Critical incident reports may well need much more narrative, written by the paramedic.

Other means, such as reports, memorandums, emails, critical incident reports, are used more within organizations to communicate, and again the key is clear, concise and accurate communication in an understandable way for the audience for whom they were intended. All of these types of written communication and the information communicated via them could be used in leadership situations to gather or disseminate information. It is important to remember that all written communication has the potential to be used as a form of evidence in a court of law, either civil or criminal. Although social media and the internet are increasingly being used as a means of communication by the NHS, ambulance services may have a website and Twitter/ Facebook accounts, but they generally are used for strategic and organization messages to be disseminated to the general public and in some cases their views obtained. However, this would need to be undertaken in accordance with professional guidance ensuring confidentiality and data protection are observed (HCPC 2012; Department of Health 2013).

Radio or telephone communication

Radio and telephone communications are a vital part of the ambulance service, as all paramedics, call handlers, dispatchers, other professionals, patients and relatives may use them at some point (Gregory and Ward 2010). These means of communication rely solely on verbal communication. Accurate, clear and concise verbal communication is vital when using them. This can make communication more challenging, because all those involved only have the words and paralinguistic features to communicate to the person on the other end of the telephone or radio. Further communication can be inhibited by poor reception or low signal strength, meaning that both parties may not hear everything the other person has said. Hence, repeating key questions or instructions would take on greater importance, to ensure all the correct information has been sent or received.

Reflection: points to consider

If you have not done so previously, try to arrange some time in ambulance call centre/control.

If you have spent time there, reflect on your experiences, in light of the theory discussed in this chapter.

- How does communication change when you cannot see the patient or the situation they are in?
- What are the specific challenges this brings?
- Just because call handlers are not *on scene*, does it make their role less valuable?
- What can student paramedics and paramedics learn from the communication style and skills seen in the ambulance control centres?

Electronic and computer-assisted communication

Technology reduces the reliance on traditional forms of communication, and there is a wide array used in the ambulance service (Gregory and Ward

2010). All of these strategies require leadership to implement and monitor their on-going effectiveness on care and the effectiveness for staff. Call handlers are able to locate caller telephone number and addresses automatically, thus aiding the speed with which a paramedic is dispatched. Paramedics will also receive some key essential information from the call centre via a mobile data terminal (MDT), however, this may not provide enough details to allow the paramedic to plan in detail what to do on arrival. This may or may not be supplemented by radio/telephone information. But the crew will be updated if the category/urgency of the call changes, via the MDT. Further computer-based systems like Advanced Medical Priority Dispatch System (AMPDS), provide the dispatcher with a protocol/ algorithm-based decision-making software, that will guide them through clinical situations by providing key questions and actions to ask the caller to undertake or respond to, until the assistance of a paramedic arrives at the scene. The accuracy of the software is completely dependent on the information provided by the caller and the skill of the call handler in communicating with the caller.

Conclusion

Communication and leadership are closely linked and significantly influence each other. Contemporary leadership is considered to be more dynamic and transformational where elements of leadership will be apparent at different levels and in various situations that occur in healthcare organizations. Therefore, it not only occurs in designated leadership roles but in the leadership behaviours of all staff. In essence, good communication is clear, concise and accurate, delivered in a sensitive way to the people involved in any situation. Leaders formulate messages, and think about how that message is sent verbally and non-verbally. Also they consider how the message might be received in any given context and can minimize misunderstanding by acknowledging each person they communicate with as an individual with individual values, beliefs and reactions to that situation. Furthermore, they actively listen to the people they communicate with. Hence, leadership and communication acknowledge the effects of socialization and social identity. The context of communication will affect the way a message is encoded, transmitted, decoded and interpreted. If good leadership is present in any situation, then there is an increased likelihood that the communication has been effective and the patient will have their concerns heard or colleagues will contribute to the organization and raise the quality of care.

Chapter key points

- Good leaders communicate well. They formulate clear messages, use appropriate verbal and non-verbal features and are consistent in applying those messages.

- Listening to others and using appropriate interpersonal skills are vital to ensure that misunderstanding and miscommunication are minimized.

- Respecting values, beliefs and cultural factors in any leadership situation is a key element of good leadership.

- Being able to tailor communication to individual leadership situations, taking into account the people involved, will potentially enhance the quality of care and organizational development.

- Repeating key messages verbally, non-verbally, in writing or electronically will help reinforce that key message.

References and suggested reading

Asterdt-Kurki, P. and Isola, A. (2001) Humour between nurse and patients, and among staff: analysis of nurses' diaries, *Journal of Advanced Nursing*, 35(3): 452–8.

Barr, J. and Dowding, L. (2012) *Leadership in Health Care*, 2nd edn. London: Sage.

Bickley, L.S. and Szilagi, P.G. (2007) Interviewing and health history, in L.S. Bickley and P.G. Szilagi (eds) *Bates Guide to Physical Examination and History Taking*. Philadelphia, PA: Lippincott Williams & Wilkins.

Blaber, A.Y. (2012) *Foundations for Paramedic Practice: A Theoretical Perspective*, 2nd edn. Maidenhead: Open University Press.

Bledsoe, B.E., Porter, R.S. and Cherry, R.A. (2010) *Essentials of Ambulance Clinician Care*, 3rd edn. Englewood Cliffs, NJ: Prentice Hall.

Cole, G.A. and Kelly, P. (2011) *Management Theory and Practice*, 7th edn. Melbourne: South-Western Cengage Learning.

Department of Health (2012) Digital strategy: leading the culture of change in health and care. Available at: http://digitalhealth.dh.gov.uk/digital-strategy (accessed 31 March 2013).

Department of Health (2013) *Patients First and Foremost: The Initial Government Response to the Report of the Mid Staffordshire NHS Foundation Trust Public Inquiry*. London: Department of Health.

Ellis, R. (2003) Defining communication, in R. Ellis, B. Gates, and N. Kenworthy (eds) *Interpersonal Communication in Nursing: Theory and Practice*, 2nd edn. Edinburgh: Churchill Livingstone, pp. 3–15.

Fellows, B. and Woolcock, M. (eds) (2009) *Nancy Caroline's Emergency Care in the Streets*, 6th edn. Philadelphia, PA: Jones and Bartlett.

Forsyth, P. (2012) *Brilliant Communication*. London: Marshall Cavendish Business.

Francis, R. (2013) *Report of the Mid Staffordshire NHS Foundation Trust Public Inquiry*. London: The Stationery Office.

Gregory, P. and Ward, A. (2010) *Saunders' Paramedic Textbook*. Edinburgh: Wiley-Blackwell.

Hartley, P. (1999) *Interpersonal Communication*, 2nd edn. London: Routledge.

HCPC (Health and Care Professions Council) (2012) *Standards of Proficiency: Paramedics*. London. HCPC.

Health and Social Care Information Centre (2012) *Data on Written Complaints in the NHS 2011–2012*. London: Health and Social Care Information Centre.

Hogg, M.A. and Vaughan, G.M. (2010) *Social Psychology*, 6th edn. Englewood Cliffs, NJ: Prentice Hall.

Kotter, J.P. (2012) *Leading Change.* Boston: Harvard Business Review Press.

Martin, J. and Swinburn, A. (2012) Paramedic clinical leadership, *Journal of Paramedic Practice*, 4(3): 181–2.

Mehrabian, A. (1981) *Silent Messages: Implicit Communication of Emotions and Attitudes,* 2nd edn. Belmont, CA: Wadsworth.

NHS Leadership Academy (2013) *Healthcare Leadership Model: The Nine Dimensions of Leadership Behaviour.* Version 1.0. Leeds: NHS Leadership Academy. Available at: www.leadershipacademy.nhs.uk/leadershipmodel (accessed 26 November 2013).

Street, P.A. (2012) Interpersonal communication: a foundation of practice, in A.Y. Blaber (ed.) *Foundation for Paramedic Practice: A Theoretical Perspective,* 2nd edn. Maidenhead: Open University Press.

Swanwick, T. and McKimm, J. (2011) *ABC of Clinical Leadership.* Chichester: Wiley-Blackwell.

Taylor, C.J. (2012) *Impact of Communication in the Healthcare Field.* Solutions Focused Consulting Group.

Taylor, J. and Armitage, E. (2012) Leadership within the ambulance service: rhetoric or reality? *Journal of Paramedic Practice*, 4(10): 564–8.

The Stationery Office (2013) *Report of the Mid Staffordshire NHS Foundation Trust Public Inquiry: Executive Summary.* London. TSO.

Twinley, R. (2012) Developing communication skills in occupational therapy and paramedic students, *Journal of Paramedic Practice*, 4(12): 705–14.

World Health Organisation (2009) *Human Factors in Patient Safety: Review of Topics and Tools.* Geneva: World Health Organisation.

Useful website

National Health Service Institute for Innovation and Improvement (2008) *Quality and service improvement tools: SBAR Situation – Background – Assessment – Recommendation.* Available at: http://www.institute.nhs.uk/quality_and_service_improvement_tools/quality (accessed 21 June 2013).

6 Working as a team
Understanding group dynamics

Marion Richardson

In this chapter

- Introduction
- Paramedics and team working
- What are teams?
- Types of teams
- Team development and group dynamics
- Team roles
- Conclusion
- Chapter key points
- References and suggested reading
- Useful websites

Introduction

Effective leadership requires individuals to work with others in teams and networks to deliver and improve healthcare services and as such *working with others* forms one of the core domains within the Leadership Framework (NHS 2011a), see Figure 6.1.

As the role of the paramedic within the National Health Service (NHS) widens to realize the recommendations of 'Taking Healthcare to the Patient: 1 and 2' (DH 2005; DH 2011) and the overarching aims of the 'Health and Social Care Act' (2012), the need for paramedics to work effectively within teams has never been more important. The wide and varied needs of patients and the variety of services required to provide their care can rarely be met by one profession and therefore it is essential that a team-working approach is adopted to ensure that patients receive high quality care (DH 2008).

Link to Chapters 1 and 3 for more detail on the Leadership Framework.

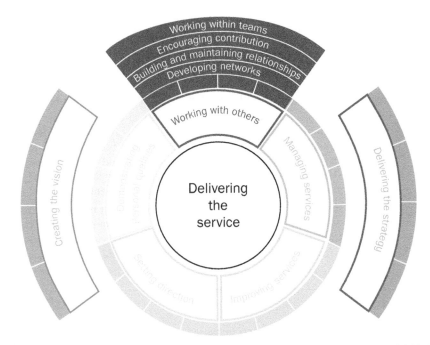

Figure 6.1 The Leadership Framework. *Source*: NHS Leadership Academy (2011a).

Paramedics and team working

The opportunities for paramedics to work with colleagues and other health professionals to improve healthcare are high, whatever their career stage or type of role they fulfil. Paramedics are now educated to make autonomous and independent decisions to manage patient care and there is an expectation that paramedics will be able to work in teams to ensure patients receive the right care, at the right place and the right time (DH 2008).

The importance of team working is clearly articulated in many influential documents that currently shape paramedic practice and includes:

- Health and Care Professions Council (HCPC) *Standards of Proficiency* (2012);
- Quality Assurance Agency (QAA) *Paramedic Benchmark Statement* (2004);
- College of Paramedics (CoP) *Paramedic Curriculum Guidance* (2013);
- the NHS Clinical Leadership Competency Framework (CLCF) (NHS 2011b);
- Healthcare Leadership Model. Version 1.0 (Leadership Academy 2013).

See Box 6.1.

Box 6.1   Various key documents that shape paramedic practice

- The QAA Paramedic Benchmark Statement (2004) promotes 'the importance of team-working and cross-professional collaboration', 'commitment to team-working', and the ability to 'operate in inter-disciplinary and inter-agency teams although these may not physically be together'.

- The Department of Health (DH 2005: 29) clearly identifies that: 'Leadership needs to focus more fully on cross-organisational teamwork, building relationships, and coaching staff to improve patient care.' '. . . effective and enhanced partnerships and teamwork with other NHS organisations, social care providers and the independent sector as crucial in order to deliver radical improvements for patients'.

- HCPC (HCPC 2012: 6–7) states that a paramedic must be able to 'contribute effectively to work undertaken as part of a multi-disciplinary team', and 'be able to work, . . . collaboratively as a member of a team'.

- CoP (CoP 2013): incorporates: 'Team-working and leadership in relation to effective team performance and reduction in human error.'

Many benefits are claimed to be associated with team working within the NHS, such as improved communication between healthcare professionals, improved coordination and service delivery, increased innovative care, enhanced contribution and timely referral between healthcare professionals, and a more holistic approach to patient care (Cooke et al. 2001, cited in Thurgood 2011; Pedler et al. 2004). On too many occasions professionals are seen to work within their own professional boundaries, not using the wealth of resources, knowledge and skill that is possessed by other professions or services within the NHS and other agencies, such as the fire service or the police force. This can lead to insular thinking, removing choice and option from patient care, thus not improving or providing the best care available. For example, reflect on the most recent child abuse case review. It does not matter which one you choose, consistently the main points are that agencies did not speak to each other. The professions worked in isolation and did not consistently share information. It is often the case that media reporting on cases focuses on the role of professionals and services. It is too easy as a society to blame the services for not realizing what was going on. It is vital to remember that the professionals in contact with the child did not perpetrate the crime of child abuse, members of the child's family did. Collaborative working, across traditional professional boundaries, and attention to detail in all communication are what will make the difference in these increasingly common stories of death by child abuse. Collaborative practice also provides paramedics with the opportunity to raise their professional status (Barrett et al. 2005), as exemplified in case study 6.1.

There is some disagreement about when inter-professional education works best. Some schools of thought recommend from the beginning of education, others prefer to wait until the individual has a sense of their own professional identity, before attempting working together. As can be seen in case study 6.1, the pre-registration students, in the last year of their course, felt both professional groups learnt so much about each other's roles and role boundaries from the day they spent together. Collaborative working can start prior to registration and seems to encourage communication, identification of difference and awareness of their own areas of expertise.

Link to Chapter 5 for more detail on the importance of communication in healthcare and its effect on clinical leadership.

Self-evaluation exercise

The NHS Leadership Academy has produced a self-assessment activity 'Working with others' that allows you to reflect on whether 'working with others' is an area you would like to develop further. It enables you to draw up an action plan targeted to your specific development needs. The self-assessment document can be accessed at: http://www.leadershipacademy.nhs.uk/wp-content/uploads/2013/03/NHSLeadership-working_with_others-20130306.pdf?29a19a.

Case study 6.1

Two groups of pre-registration students were invited to the flexible learning environment within the university campus. This area is a fully functional flat that has been equipped with cameras, sound systems, access to personal microphones, recording equipment and a room where students can observe the scenario live and then can play back specific points for discussion at any time.

The students were 3rd year student paramedics and midwives. The lecturers had worked together to create scenarios for the day and there were many props, including ones to discharge large volumes of blood, simulating large volume haemorrhage.

After working together in simulation for the day, the two groups had developed some appreciation of the others' role and role boundaries. Both groups relayed stories from practice where they had felt the paramedic or midwife was being obstructive, but when they discussed the issues, it was often the case that the professional was bound by protocol or policy and it was not a case of being awkward or obstructive at all. The lack of clear communication was an issue in many of the cases.

One of the most fundamental problems encountered by the student midwives was the lack of understanding about the paramedic uniform. They believed all personnel in green uniforms were paramedics, and had the same skill set. This is a common misconception among the general public and obviously among other professional groups too. Considering this most fundamental issue, it is easy to appreciate why other professionals or services may think that an individual is being obstructive, rather than appreciating the various levels of staff within the ambulance service. Perhaps this is something for the profession to consider. Individually, would you now consider being clearer about who you are and what you can or cannot do when you meet other professionals at a call?

What are teams?

It may be beneficial at this point to explore the definition of a team and the types of teams that we may encounter. Teams historically are associated with providing additional strength or power, e.g. a team of huskies pulling a sledge (Colenso 1997). It is this 'synergy', where the efforts of the whole are greater than the sum of the individual parts, which has led to the increased emphasis on team working to enhance performance within the NHS (Colenso 1997; DH 2011).

'Team' is a term or sometimes a convenient label that is often used to describe people working together and countless definitions of 'teams' within healthcare exist, e.g. Payne (2000) identified 15 definitions of 'teams', and what is meant and understood by this term varies enormously (Bleakley 2013). It is not the aim of this chapter to debate the appropriateness of the terminology used, what is important is that the characteristics that enable people to work effectively together are identified. To clarify what is meant by 'team' in this chapter Katzenbach and Smith's (1993: 45) definition is used:

> A team is a small number of people with complementary skills who are committed to a common purpose, performance goals and approach for which they hold themselves mutually accountable.

It is clear that 'effective' teams are more than just groups of people working together. While a team can be described as a group of people, not all groups can be described as teams, and there are several common characteristics that are seen to distinguish teams from groups which are identified in Table 6.1.

Gorman (1998) and Katzenbach and Smith (1993) suggest several basic elements that are necessary for an effective team:

- A small number of team members: there is little agreement as to what constitutes a 'small' team but for practical purposes a small team consists of between two and 20 members. This is usually the case in ambulance services, with traditional crews of two people. When the situation warrants, teams come together to be able to cope with more than one casualty. Solo responders often work with the teams of two colleagues,

Table 6.1   Characteristics of groups and teams

Groups	Teams
Members have individual accountability but leader takes overall responsibility.	Members have individual and collective responsibility for achieving outcomes. Members are dependent on each other to achieve the final result.
On the whole, members work independently but come together to exchange information and perspectives.	Members are interdependent and frequently engage in discussion, decision-making, problem-solving, and planning.
Members focus on their individual goals, outcomes and challenges.	Committed to common purpose and shared goals.
Members are able to define their individual roles, responsibilities, and tasks but are not involved in the planning of objectives.	Members have a clear understanding of their own and each other's roles and responsibilities. Members have a sense of ownership.
Work is allocated to group members and members make their contribution without concern for what others need to achieve.	Team leaders and members collaboratively agree goals and approach to work and develop effective communication strategies.
Members' skills may be random.	Members have complementary skills and make different contributions towards a common goal including technical and functional expertise; problem solving and interpersonal skills.

Source: Adapted from: Brounstein (2002); Payne (2000); and Katzenbach and Smith (1993).

especially when the patient requires transportation. The key factor is not so much about numbers but the availability of members to engage in face-to-face interaction (Shaw 1981, cited in Hargie et al. 1994).

- Team members have defined roles and complementary skills including:
  - technical or functional expertise;
  - problem solving and decision-making skills;
  - interpersonal skills.
- Interaction between members: communication between members is essential to unite the team, to organize themselves; to pool resources and problem-solve to cooperatively reach the teams goals.
- The team should have a common purpose and performance goals.
- A common working approach.
- Team members should be mutually accountable for achieving shared goals and outcomes.
- Team identity and a sense of belonging.

It is apparent from the above that there are many organizational units within the NHS that are called teams but lack many of the features of a team, for example, radiographers work in a department, but consistently work alone, as do phlebotomists. However, if you asked both of these groups of people if they worked in a team, they would probably classify the fellow radiographers and phlebotomists as their team of co-workers whom they meet at the start and the end of each day (Gorman 1998; Katzenbach and Smith 1993). As Pedler et al. (2004) point out, however, many tasks can be successfully achieved by appropriate allocation of work to individuals or carried out by a group working cooperatively. For some jobs, getting together to share information and tasks and make simple decisions does not require the full interdependent collaborative working of a 'true team'. However, for more difficult or uncertain situations, the high collaboration and interdependence of an effective team are required. Understanding the fundamental differences between groups and teams will enable paramedics to work within or lead a team more effectively and give insight into how to strengthen team working in their area of practice.

Reflection: points to consider

- Think about two situations that have required more than three ambulance paramedics to be in attendance. One situation where the team working was good and effective, and one where the team working was poor and lacked effect.
- Reflect on the team working that went on, did the teams work well together? If not, why might that have been?
- Think of a time when a larger team worked well together, what do you think were the reasons for this success?
- List what you think are the keys to successful team working in the paramedic profession.

Types of teams

It is important for paramedics to have an accurate understanding of the types of working that occur between healthcare professionals, as can be seen by reading case study 6.1. A review of the literature shows that the concept of working together within healthcare can be confusing with a variety of terms being used to describe what appears to be very similar activities e.g. *multi-disciplinary, inter-disciplinary, inter-agency* and *inter-professional*, which is further complicated by associated relationships described as team working, collaboration and partnership (Barrett et al. 2005; West 2012). Such terminology appears frequently in key documents, guidelines and job descriptions relevant to paramedic practice and is sometimes used interchangeably; however, these terms have different implications for practice (HCPC 2000; QAA 2004; CoP 2013; Payne 2000).

Table 6.2 Terminology used to describe working with others

Term	Definition
Prefixes	
Multi	The term *multi* suggests that several organizational or professional groups contribute to the team. Members, however, work within their own professional or organizational boundaries within the team and do not need to adapt their knowledge and skills to accommodate their team role.
Inter	*Inter* implies joint working between members of two or more professions. This relationship implies that some adaptation of professional roles, knowledge, skills and responsibilities is required to interact with other professional groups or agencies within the team.
Trans	*Trans* suggests that professionals cross disciplinary boundaries and take on and engage in activities usually associated with another professional group. In trans-disciplinary working, information, knowledge and skills are transferred across disciplinary boundaries.
Adjectives	
Agency	An organization that provides a particular service, e.g. the ambulance service, the Fire and Rescue Service and the Police.
Professional	Membership of the team is limited to members who are regulated by a professional or regulating body, e.g. HCPC.
Disciplinary	The term *disciplinary* suggests a specific branch or field of practice, associated with specialist professional roles or a subspecialty within a profession.
Relationship	
Collaboration	Collaboration infers the working together of more or less equal partners to achieve something that neither member could achieve alone or *synergy*.
Partnership	Partnerships are mutually beneficial to each member.
Team work	Team work is a cooperative effort by the members of a group or team to achieve a common goal.

Source: Adapted from: Payne (2000: 9); Day (2006); and Kvarnström (2008).

Table 6.2 shows a range of frequently encountered prefixes, adjectives and relationships, and seeks to clarify the terminology used to describe working with others.

Sporting analogies of different types of teams and links to paramedic practice

Payne (2000) describes a series of useful sporting analogies to explain the different kinds of teams that exist within the healthcare setting: the football team, the tennis team and the athletics team. These analogies are interesting and when we look closer at how these teams work, we can identify some of the challenges that paramedics will face when working within healthcare teams.

- *The football team*: All players within a football team have a strong identity and practise frequently together. Members play together at the same time on a pitch and interact throughout the match and they win or lose as a team (Payne 2000). Paramedics may liken this type of team to the consultant-led specialist trauma teams within major trauma centres. Typically, a team of this kind has dedicated team members, consisting of a full range of trauma specialists who have shared objectives and a strong team identity. All team members are present throughout the treatment of the patient which allows for instantaneous communication within the team and access to specialist treatment. The roles of the trauma specialists and support staff within the team are clearly defined and because trauma cases are frequently directed to such units, the members frequently practise together (Gorman 1998; South Tees Hospital Foundation Trust 2013). This type of team has *collective responsibility* (Øvretveit 1997: 77) and that clearly meets the basic elements of an effective team described earlier.

- *The tennis team*: In the tennis team each individual plays separately and has to win their match. However, all members do the same thing and *play tennis* (Payne 2000: 8). Paramedics working in an Ambulance Trust are an example of this type of team. Unlike the trauma team above, the team are not all present at the same time. The size of the team in this case is large and as the numbers of members in a team increase, the identity of the team becomes blurred and the identity of the organization takes over (Gorman 1998). Several aspects of this type of team make it difficult to meet the basic elements of an effective team, e.g. the large size of the team weakens mutual accountability for achieving shared aims, and objectives become weakened as individuals and subgroups take responsibility for their own *piece of the jigsaw* of care, rather than functioning as a single team (Gorman 1998; Katzenbach and Smith 1993).

- *The athletics team*: All team members of an athletics team compete separately and do different things and this is synonymous to a multi-professional team where each professional carries out their role and is accountable to their professional or organizational hierarchy (Payne 2000). Professionals within the multi-professional team refer work to each other and are influenced by each other's ideas, e.g. paramedics working within a primary healthcare team. This *coordinated* team typically consists of a large number of members who look after a wide range of patients, who are widely dispersed. While members have individual professional roles, these are sometimes blurred as several skills within this type of team are common to all healthcare professionals. Patients are usually seen by one member of the team at a time and some patients may see several members of the team in any one day; some members of the team may not see the patient at all. This type of team may find it difficult to meet and communication between members can be difficult (Katzenbach and Smith 1993). While each member may have individual specific goals, their shared objective is loosely defined. There is a general expectation that teams are cohesive and integrated but this is difficult to achieve in large teams of this type where communication is difficult and the size of the team impedes team building, a sense of belonging, and co-ownership (Gorman 1998).

Teams within the NHS

Within the NHS, great emphasis is increasingly being placed on developing multi- and inter-disciplinary team working. A major national study of team working carried out by the Healthcare Team Effectiveness Project concluded that team working is essential to ensure the efficient delivery of high quality care (Jones and Jenkins 2007). Multi-professional, multi-disciplinary and multi-agency working brings together and utilizes the knowledge, skills and expertise of a variety of different professional groups to provide a structured approach to healthcare delivery. See Box 6.2 for ambulance-specific examples. In a multi-professional team, professionals are not required to adapt their professional role, knowledge base, skill set or agency responsibilities while working within the team. Conversely in inter-professional, inter-disciplinary and inter-agency working, professionals are usually required to adapt their role and develop their knowledge and skills base in order to effectively operate as a member of the team, cross disciplinary boundaries and take on roles traditionally associated with other professionals (Payne 2000). Trans-disciplinary team work involves transfer of knowledge and skills across disciplinary boundaries and ultimately leads to professionals taking on roles usually associated with other professional groups.

Box 6.2   Examples of paramedics working within teams

- *Multidisciplinary team*: Community paramedics within the North East Ambulance Service NHS Foundation Trust work within a primary care team of nurses and General Practitioners (GPs) to provide a more dynamic and proactive service than the traditional blue-light service which existed previously (NHS 2011). Paramedics have several skills that overlap with those of the nurses and GPs, e.g. interacting with and assessing patients, treating illness and negotiating care plans. By blurring the traditional boundaries of the healthcare professionals within the primary care team, patients are able to remain in their own home and unnecessary admissions to hospital are avoided. Additional benefits of such arrangements include improved record keeping and communication between team members of the primary care team, the provision of timely appropriate treatment and continuity of patient care (Thurgood 2011).

- *Clinical advice paramedics* (hear and treat) promote cohesive working and teamwork by engaging proactively with control service staff, frontline paramedics and other healthcare professionals such as district nurses and General Practitioners to ensure that the most appropriate care pathway is accessed to meet individual patient needs. Hear and treat paramedics are usually based in ambulance control. Consequently, they usually do not ever meet the patient face to face, but are influential in the direct care the patient receives from other members of the team. See the profile of the clinical advice paramedic for more detail.

- *Working within a multi-agency/inter-agency team*: The Department of Health Emergency Preparedness Division (DH EPD) started the Ambulance Hazardous Area Response Teams (HART) programme in 2005. HARTs are specially trained and equipped ambulance clinicians who attend incidents involving a chemical, biological, radiological, nuclear or explosive (CBRNE) element. They work as part of a team consisting of police and fire service colleagues in the high risk *inner cordon* during hazardous incidents. The Department of Health (2011) refers to HART teams as *multi-agency teams*, however, it could be argued that this type of team is more accurately described as an inter-agency team as adaptations to the paramedic's role, knowledge and skills base have been necessary to enable them to interact with the roles of other agencies.

The nature of paramedic practice requires that paramedics work within a wide variety of teams (see Box 6.2) that may not be physically located together, and that are dependent on the diverse needs of their patients. For the paramedic, team working ranges from tightly knit units such as members of a regular crew to 'loosely woven' situations that emerge to meet specific needs of individual patients or situations (multi-disciplinary or multi-agency). Teams may collaborate with each other in practice or individual members may work alone on behalf of the team, e.g. Specialist paramedics may work alone on a rapid response vehicle but they are very much part of a team that supports operational staff and engages in multi-disciplinary team (MDT) working. Indeed, the Specialist paramedic profile 5 (paramedic practitioner B) at the beginning of the book, has *multi-disciplinary working with a range of other health and social care professionals, such as GPs, nurses and social care workers and collaborative decision making,* as part of their job description. The paramedic practitioner profile states the post holder should *Liaise with other agencies and disciplines, promote and develop cross-trust partnership working.*

Teams within health and social care may also be defined by their membership, their function or their area of clinical responsibility (Thurgood 2011), e.g. mental health teams and hazard area response teams (HART), which have a specified structure and objectives (Barrett et al. 2005). A team may also be a convenient way to describe a group of staff with a common manager and role, e.g. a divisional team.

Team development and group dynamics

As previously mentioned, teams are more than merely groups of people working together. It is widely agreed that groups go through a number of predictable stages as they develop into an effective team and several theoretical models exist that support this notion (Smith 2005). Arguably one of the most commonly used and influential frameworks is 'Tuckman's model of group development'. This framework gives a helpful explanation of the five stages of team development and behaviour. Tuckman's work identified that most groups experience the same developmental stages and experience similar conflicts and issues throughout their lifespan. It is how these issues are resolved that determines the success of the group completing the task (Smith 2005). Awareness of the characteristics of each stage of development that teams go through can enable team leaders and members of the group to explain the behaviour of the group in the context of team development and adopt strategies to effectively manage each stage (Colenso 1997). Sometimes teams who are 'stuck' revert back to previous stages of group development, and if this is recognized, then strategies can be employed to get the group back on track.

Tuckman's model of group development has the following five stages:

1. forming
2. storming
3. norming
4. performing
5. adjourning.

Forming

As the title suggests, this is the initial coming together of a group (though as mentioned earlier, a group may return to this stage following change, e.g. the introduction of a new group member). During this stage of group development, members are likely to try to get to know each other and avoid controversy in an attempt to be accepted by the team (Day 2006). Often at this point individual members may not fully understand their role and feel anxious about how the group will work, which may lead to members 'testing' the processes of the team and the team leader. It is important at this point that the team leader is able to identify the strengths and weaknesses of members of the group to be able to identify how their skills can contribute to the task in hand. The team leader's role in this stage of team development is to get all of the team members on board by creating a compelling and attractive vision of what is possible for the team to achieve (Colenso 1997). The group needs to define the team's objectives and how the group is going to achieve them. This can be a very stressful time for the team leader. Colenso (1997) suggests that during this stage of development the behaviour that is observed is that of a group of individuals rather than team behaviour which emerges in the next two stages *storming* and *norming*.

Storming

During this *stormy* but necessary stage of group development, team members will challenge each other, question issues such as worth and feasibility of the objectives and seek to clarify who is responsible for what (Day 2006). During the *storming stage*, characterized by conflict, struggles for power may occur and some individuals may try to assert themselves and challenge the guidance and direction of the leader, others will try to establish their *niche* within the team. This unsettling stage may result in non-engagement of some members while others attempt to dominate. At this point there may still be uncertainty of roles and the team leader needs to ensure that the team purpose and the roles that members play within the team are clarified.

Storming enables the team to begin to establish a common set of values and objectives. While this stage is uncomfortable for team leaders and members alike, it is necessary to establish an effective team. During the storming process the morale of the team may be low and individuals may lose confidence and it is at this stage that teams are most likely to fail. An understanding that this is a natural stage of team development will help the team progress to the next stage.

Norming

To move from *storming* to *norming*, conflict within the group must be replaced by listening to each other and problem solving (Day 2006). *Norming* marks the stage when the individual roles of members are recognized and the boundaries established and the team starts to function in harmony, e.g. the student paramedic will develop an understanding of the boundaries and expectations of their role and that of the paramedic in the delivery of patient care. The contribution of each member is valued and any preconceived opinions give way to ideas based on facts presented by team members. It is during the norming stage that the team is very creative. This is facilitated by constructive feedback and exploration of ideas related to the objectives of the team. The leader should adopt the role of facilitator at this stage and empower the team to take on the delegated tasks. In this stage a form of self-regulation emerges to enable the team to function and survive and this is achieved by the development of informal rules of behaviour that are shared and enforced by members of the team (Thompson 2011).

Performing

During this stage the team works efficiently towards the team's objectives and is at its most effective and *performing*. Team members work harmoniously together, are motivated and successful. Members are aware of their role in the team and the contribution they make in achieving the team's objectives. At this stage in the lifecycle of the team the leader oversees the work of the team, trusting them to act on the tasks and within the roles allocated to them (Ellis and Abbott 2013).

Adjourning

Adjourning marks an end or change in the team's working life. This may be a result of achievement of objectives, changes to team composition, or changes in tasks that affect the group dynamics of a team. Successful teams who attain their objectives and where their work is finished can experience sadness and members may *mourn* the end of the team.

Reflection: points to consider

You are about to meet a new group of people on a course lasting several months. Think about the stages of group development and see if over time, you can identify any of the five stages.

The range of professional groups from which teams are formed within pre-hospital and out-of-hospital care generally remains fairly static. However, the combination of professional groups required to meet individual patient needs and the individuals who represent those various professions frequently changes. Change of membership within any team will affect the group dynamics and may cause the team to revert back to previous stages of Tuckman's model. The introduction of new members to the team is not always a negative event and may well lead to stronger development of the team.

Team roles

It is fairly easy to identify the professional roles of the different members within a multidisciplinary team or roles that are linked to skill mix, e.g. a crew consisting of an emergency care supporter and paramedic or roles within a hierarchy, e.g. Director of Operations and operations manager. However, members of a team will also have 'team roles' in addition to their professional or occupational roles. It is important to distinguish someone's professional or occupational role from their *team role*. The significance of this is that the 'professional or occupational role' of people appointed to a given job should be the same, e.g. paramedics with the same skill set share the same functional role, however, each paramedic within a given team may adopt very different *team roles* which are concerned with group relations rather than the function that the team has to perform (Payne 2000). A balance between team roles within a team and how team members interact with each other has a crucial impact on effective team working (Belbin 2010b; Bach and Ellis 2011).

Team role theory

There are many contributors to team role theory. Benne and Skeats' team roles were derived from the study of group dynamics. They divided team roles into three categories: (1) those that fulfil group tasks; (2) those that maintain group cohesion; and, finally, (3) those that relate to the personality and pursuit of personal needs of the individual (cited in Payne 2000). Belbin (1981) identified eight team roles to which he later added a ninth role that individual members can play during a team's life, which he categorized into three main groups: (1) action-orientated roles; (2) people-orientated roles; and (3) cerebral roles (Belbin 1981; Belbin 2010a; Day 2006). Subsequently in 2009, Sullivan and Decker suggested that individual roles can be grouped into two categories: (1) *task roles* that focus on the team's objectives and function; and (2) *nurturing roles* that are concerned with maintaining the interpersonal needs of the team (cited in Bach and Ellis 2011). All of these theories bear similarities to the early work of Benne and Skeats, suggesting that a well-established and consistent view of team roles has been established.

In healthcare there is usually no formal selection of team members based on their 'team roles', however, analysis of teams in relation to team roles arguably can lead to improved problem solving and more efficient performance (Thurgood 2011). Belbin continues to be one of the major contributors to team role theory (see Table 6.3). A team role, according to Belbin, is the characteristic manner in which a team member interacts with other members of the team facilitating the progress of the team as a whole (Belbin 2010). Belbin argues that successful teams will have all or most of the roles within it. If significant roles are missing, the team will be unbalanced and will function less effectively. Most people have main and secondary roles and the roles they adopt within a team will be dependent on the roles taken on by others.

Belbin's team roles do not refer to the personality of team members but the behavioural characteristics that people can display when working together in teams. An understanding of these roles will enable you to recognize the contributions that you and your colleagues make to the team and will enhance the way you work together. For example, on an ambulance station there may be 10 paramedics, all with the same clinical skills. Their role within the station team will vary, some will demonstrate the characteristics of the role of co-ordinator, implementer, team-worker. As the team develops, roles will generally become clearer and more defined. Your team role may vary according to the team in which you are involved, as your role will be dependent on who else is in the team and the team's objectives. You may need to forego using your *preferred* team role and adopt what Belbin refers to as a *manageable role* which we can assume if required, e.g. if there is a lack of a desired role within the team or because another person is already operating in your preferred role, this is referred to as 'making a team role sacrifice' (Belbin 2010b). Role sacrifice is possible because most people tend to display more than one preferred role, and this also means that a relatively small team could quite easily represent all of Belbin's team roles.

In addition to preferred and manageable roles, we all have 'least preferred' roles. Belbin advises that team members should not assume these roles, as working against role type requires great effort which will likely result in poor outcomes (Belbin 2010b). Each team role also has an associated weakness which is allowable in the team because of the strength which goes with it.

Reflection: points to consider

- Many ambulance services are using stand-by points, as an attempt to meet stringent government response targets. What effect might this have on team working?
- In some areas, smaller ambulance stations are being closed and in their place are large, super-stations, covering a huge geographical area. What may be the implications for paramedic teams who are organized into these super-stations?

Working in a team is common in any working environment. Sometimes teams are cohesive, efficient and produce high quality work, sometimes they are the direct opposite. The theory surrounding teamwork and team roles is important to consider, in an attempt to examine and make sense of your own experiences.

Table 6.3 Belbin's team roles

Role	Typical features	Role description	Allowable weaknesses
Action Orientated roles			
Shaper	Shapers are highly motivated, assertive and dynamic individuals. May be highly strung.	Shapers thrive on pressure and are driven by achievement. They 'shape the way in which the team effort is applied' (Belbin 1981: 168) and will challenge team inertia or ineffectiveness. Shapers have the drive and courage to overcome obstacles.	Shapers tend to be argumentative and are prone to irritation and impatience. They can provoke others and may hurt other members' feelings.
Implementer	Implementers are conservative, loyal, practicable and predictable. They are hard-working, self-disciplined, and driven by common sense.	Implementers are able to systematically organize concepts and plans into practical actions.	Implementers can lack flexibility, be unresponsive to new unproven ideas and resistant to change.
Completer-Finisher	Completer-Finishers are meticulous, organized, hard-working, but often anxious.	Completer-Finishers are quality and schedule driven. They show great attention to detail, are highly accurate and search out errors and omissions. They have a capacity to follow through, achieve perfection and deliver on time.	Completer-Finishers have a tendency to worry unnecessarily about small things, tend to nit-pick and find it difficult to delegate. Their anxiousness may inhibit the team.

Category	Role	Characteristics	Contribution	Allowable weaknesses
People Orientated Roles	Co-ordinator	Co-ordinators are mature, calm, self-confident and controlled.	Co-ordinators welcome all contributions on their merits without prejudice. They have a strong sense of the objectives to be achieved and delegate work to others.	Co-ordinators can delegate too much personal work away and can be seen as manipulative. Co-ordinators tend to be ordinary in terms of intellect and creativity.
	Resource Investigator	Resource Investigators are 'extroverted, enthusiastic, curious' (Belbin 1981:78) and good communicators.	Resource Investigators are good networkers who are able to develop new contacts and explore and report on new ideas, developments and resources external to the group. They borrow and develop ideas rather than initiate ideas. Resource Investigators have 'an ability to respond to challenge' (Belbin 1981:78).	Resource Investigators may lose interest following the initial challenge, have a tendency to be overoptimistic and can be lazy.
	Team-worker	Team-workers are 'socially orientated' (Belbin 1981: 78), cooperative, sensitive, perceptive and diplomatic.	Team-workers are very supportive and sociable and are good listeners. They are perceptive and respond to people and situations to uphold team spirit and provide a calming influence.	Team-workers tend to be 'indecisive at moments of crisis' (Belbin 1981: 78) and tend not to commit during decision-making.
Cerebral Roles	Plant	Plants display genius, imagination, intellect and knowledge. They are 'individualistic, serious minded and unorthodox' (Belbin 1981:78).	Plants are creative and original and excel in 'advancing new ideas and strategies and pay special attention to major issues' (Belbin 2010: 183). They tend to be imaginative and unorthodox when looking for ways to approach difficult problems facing the team.	Plants find criticism hard. They are often introverted, preferring to work alone. They tend to 'disregard practical detail and protocols' (Belbin 1981: 78). They are often too preoccupied to communicate effectively.
	Monitor Evaluator	Monitor Evaluators tend to be serious, unemotional, and prudent. They think strategically and exhibit discretion and hard-headedness (Payne 2000: 121).	Monitor Evaluators critically analyse all options and suggestions so the team is better placed to achieve a balanced impartial and well considered, accurate judgement.	Monitor Evaluators often lack drive and inspiration and as poor motivators may be considered boring. They may be thought of as unemotional. Monitor Evaluators tend to be reactive not proactive.
	Specialist	Specialists tend to be single-minded, self-starting, and dedicated.	Specialists bring knowledge and skills to the team that are in rare supply. Specialists are experts who are dedicated to their own subject and prefer to contribute to the team only in this area. They are driven by standards.	The contribution to the team by specialists may be limited and may dwell on technicalities. Their preoccupation with their specialism may be at the expense of the team's bigger picture. May not care for teamwork.

Source: Adapted from: Ellis and Abbott (2013); Belbin (1981, 2013, 2010a, 2010b), Payne (2000); and Burton and Ormond (2011).

Conclusion

Without doubt it is clear that working in teams in healthcare is important to ensure high quality care. The nature of pre- and out-of-hospital care requires that paramedics can work effectively in a wide range of teams that form in response to patients' needs. Several key areas have emerged from the literature that will support effective team working whether this is in a crew or working as part of a large team that is not located together: a clear understanding of one's own role and the role of others within the team, a common goal and an effective system of communication.

It is recognized that many organizational units operating within the NHS are called teams but lack some of the basic features and characteristics of a team and this will create challenges for paramedics to ensure effective team working is achieved. Understanding the characteristics of teams, their developmental stages and roles within a team will enhance working practices.

Chapter key points

- Working with others is a core domain in the Leadership Framework.
- Paramedics must work effectively in a range of teams to ensure patients receive the right care, in the right place and at the right time.
- Effective teams are more than groups of people working together.
- Working in healthcare teams can take many forms.
- Team development follows predictable stages.
- Understanding team roles will enable you to recognize your contribution and that of your colleagues to the success of the team.

References and suggested reading

Bach, S. and Ellis, P. (2011) *Leadership, Management and Team Working in Nursing.* Exeter: Learning Matters Ltd.

Barrett, G., Sellman, D. and Thomas, J. (eds) (2005) *Inter-Professional Working in Health and Social Care: Professional Perspectives.* Basingstoke: Palgrave Macmillan.

Belbin, R.M. (1981) *Management Teams: Why They Succeed Or Fail.* Oxford: Butterworth-Heinemann Ltd.

Belbin, R.M. (2010a) *Management Teams: Why They Succeed Or Fail,* 3rd edn. Oxford: Elsevier.

Belbin, R.M. (2010b) *Team Roles at Work,* 2nd edn. Oxford: Elsevier.

Bleakley, A. (2013) Working in 'teams' in an era of 'liquid' healthcare: what is the use of theory? *Journal of Inter-professional Care,* 27:18–26.

Brounstein, M. (2002) *Managing Teams for Dummies.* New York: Wiley Publishing Ltd.

Burton, R. and Ormond, G. (eds) (2011) *Nursing: Transition to Professional Practice.* Oxford: Oxford University Press.

Colenso, M. (1997) *High Performing Teams in Brief.* Oxford: Butterworth-Heinemann.

College of Paramedics (2013) *Paramedic Curriculum Guidance,* 3rd edn. Bridgwater: College of Paramedics.

Day, J. (2006) *Expanding Nursing and Healthcare Practice: Inter-Professional Working.* Cheltenham: Nelson Thornes Ltd.

DH (Department of Health) (1998) *Modernising Social Services: Quality in the NHS.* London: HMSO.

DH (Department of Health) (2005) *Taking Healthcare to the Patient: Transforming NHS Ambulance Services.* London: HMSO.

DH (Department of Health) (2008) *High Quality Care for All: NHS Next Stage Review: Final Report.* London: HMSO.

DH (Department of Health) (2011) *Taking Healthcare to the Patient 2: A Review of 6 Years' Progress and Recommendations for the Future.* London: Association of Ambulance Chief Executives.

Ellis, P. and Abbott, J. (2013) What new leaders need to understand about their teams, *British Journal of Cardiac Nursing,* 8(1): 44–8.

Gorman, P. (1998) *Managing Multi-Disciplinary Teams in the NHS.* London: Kogan Page Limited.

Hargie, O., Saunders, C. and Dickson, D. (1994) *Social Skills in Inter-Personal Communication,* 3rd edn. London: Routledge.

HCPC (Health and Care Professions Council) (2012) *Standards of Proficiency - Paramedics.* London: Health and Care Professions Council.

HM Coroner (2011) *Inquest into the London Bombings of 7ᵗʰ July 2005.* London: The Stationary Office.

House of Commons Health Committee (2003) *The Victoria Climbié Inquiry Report.* London: The Stationery Office.

House of Commons Health Committee (2009) *The Protection of Children in England: A Progress Report.* London: The Stationery Office.

Jones, R. and Jenkins, F. (eds) (2007) *Key Topics in Healthcare Management: Understanding the Big Picture.* Oxford: Radcliffe Publishing.

Johnson, D.W. and Johnson, F.P. (2009) *Joining Together: Group Theory and Group Skills,* 10th edn. Harlow: Pearson.

Katzenbach, J.R. (1998) *Teams at the Top: Unleashing the Potential of Both Teams and Individual Leaders.* Boston: Harvard Business School Press.

Katzenbach, J.R. and Smith, D.K. (1993) *The Wisdom of Teams: Creating the High Performance Organisation.* London: McGraw-Hill.

Kvarnström, S. (2008) Difficulties in collaboration: a critical incident study of inter-professional healthcare teamwork, *Journal of Inter-Professional Care,* 22(2): 191–203.

NHS Leadership Academy (2011a) *Leadership Framework.* Coventry: NHS Institute for Innovation and Improvement.

NHS Leadership Academy (2011b) *Clinical Leadership Competency Framework.* Coventry: NHS Institute for Innovation and Improvement.

NHS Leadership Academy (2013) *Healthcare Leadership Model: The Nine Dimensions of Leadership Behaviour.* Version 1.0. Leeds: NHS Leadership Academy. Available at: www.leadershipacademy.nhs.uk/leadershipmodel (accessed 26 November 2013).

NHS Ambulance Chief Executive Group (2009) *Report of the National Steering Group on Clinical Leadership in the Ambulance Service.* London: The Stationery Office.

Øvreveit, J. (1993) *Coordinating Community Care.* Buckingham: Open University Press.

Payne, M. (2000) *Teamwork in Multi-Professional Care.* Basingstoke: Palgrave.

Pedler, M., Burgoyne, J. and Boydell, T. (2004) *A Manager's Guide to Leadership*. Maidenhead: McGraw-Hill Professional.

Quality Assurance Agency (QAA) for Higher Education (2004) *Benchmark Statement for Paramedic Science*. Gloucester. QAA. Available at: www.qaa.ac.uk/academicinfrastructure/benchmark/health/Paramedicscience.pdf (accessed May 2013).

Smith, M.K. (2005) Bruce W. Tuckman: forming, storming, norming and performing in groups, in *The Encyclopaedia of Informal Education*. Available at: www.infed.org/thinkers/ tuckman.htm (accessed 29 January 2013).

South Tees Hospitals NHS Foundation Trust (2013) *Major Trauma Centre*. Available at: http://www.southtees.nhs.uk/services/accident-and-emergency/major-trauma-centre/9 (accessed 24 September 2013).

NHS Modernisation Agency (2004) *The ECP Report: Right Skill, Right Time, Right Place*. London: Department of Health.

The Stationery Office (2012) *The Health and Social Care Act*. London: The Stationery Office.

Thompson, L.L. (2011) *Making the Team: A Guide for Managers*, 2nd edn. Harlow: Pearson Education.

Thurgood, G. (2011) Teamwork: working with other people, in R. Burton and G. Ormond (eds) *Nursing: Transition to Professional Practice*. Oxford: Oxford University Press, pp. 118–57.

West, M.A. (2012) *Effective Teamwork: Practical Lessons from Organizational Research*. Chichester: John Wiley and Sons Ltd.

Useful websites

Belbin team roles
http://www.belbin.com.
Leadership academy
http://www.leadershipacademy.nhs.uk/discover/leadership-framework/.

7 Decision-making

Paul Jones

Introduction

This chapter will consider the paramedic's ability to make decisions as a leader. The main focus will be on decision-making as a concept, problem solving and theories or styles of decision-making. There is no getting away from it, good leaders make decisions. Whether those decisions are good in their own right, or not, is a topic which is open to debate and opinion. It needs to be realized nonetheless that the key is in making the decision in the first place. The worst form of decision is indecision.

Many decisions can be carefully planned before the actions involved are executed, but in paramedic practice this is not always the case and the decisions that are made have to be relatively *dynamic*. These dynamic decision-making moments are what can make the paramedic profession so attractive to so many. The process involves the linking of many factors and then establishing a form of judgement about what actions need to be taken. In practice this makes the clinician (in this case the paramedic) accountable for the quality, safety and effectiveness of their chosen actions (NMC 2010).

The National Health Service (NHS) Leadership Academy (Leadership Academy 2011) suggests that leaders make decisions based on a number of factors, predominantly their own personal and professional values and the evidence that is available to them at the time. Values can include service, reverence, integrity, wisdom, dedication and (where appropriate) even creativity (St. Mary's Healthcare 2013). Evidence – which can be defined as information used to support reasoning, judgement or decisions – can and does include observations, policy and research. But in the real-time world of paramedic practice, there is a risk of that evidence in whatever form it takes becoming blurred. Nevertheless, it is the combination of these factors which defines or determines how good the final decision is. If the leader's own values are questionable, then the chances are that the decisions that they make will be questionable too, if the evidence available to them is poor, then there is a high probability that the decisions that they make will be poor too. It is with this in mind that paramedics are reminded that they are always at risk of making clinical decisions that will not be good ones – decisions which are not based on values or evidence but based on rules and poor quality evidence (the only evidence available at the time to work with). The evidence in question may be higher-level evidence which has guided protocol or alternatively circumstantial evidence at the scene of an incident with which they are working.

Modern leaders who work to high professional standards not only engage in the delivery of care. Paramedics (see Figure 7.1) all have a responsibility to shape Trust decision-making processes in order to benefit the needs of the profession, the Trust and the patients that they serve. The joint shaping of

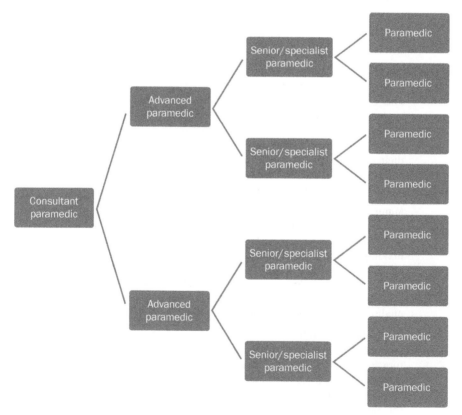

Figure 7.1   Example of paramedic leadership structure.

these processes allows consistent application of positive values and assists in the education of key players at all levels. The 2013 Francis Report highlights the issue of leadership and culture within the NHS. It asks the question: why were the leaders blind and deaf to the feedback they received from frontline staff, patients and families (*The Guardian* Online 2013)?

Case study 7.1

A patient has suffered from cardiac arrest and it is decided that intravenous (IV) access is needed in order that drugs can be delivered. Unfortunately, the paramedic on scene has difficulty siting an IV so decides to call for the assistance of a Senior paramedic to site an intraosseous needle. This is performed to good effect and the patient has appropriate drugs delivered via an appropriate route to good effect. Following this, the events and subsequent decisions are reviewed by an Advanced paramedic and a process of 360° feedback is engaged in for reflective purposes focusing mainly on the decisions made by the clinicians at the scene and the alternatives available to them.

Link to Chapter 4 to read more about organizational culture.

Further to making decisions themselves, a good paramedic leader should also have the capability to empower others, offering opportunity for engagement of all in the decision-making process. Shared decision-making is seen as being the crux of patient-centred care and is a key ingredient to improving quality in healthcare (Godolphin 2009). This can be achieved by respecting expertise and managing differences in opinion in order to work towards a final consensus. In doing this, however, the leader has to ensure that they continue to lead and not be led. There is the risk of over-empowerment to consider, paramedic leaders' decision-making needs to remain rigorous while considering all factors – external and internal – to the Trust that employs and governs them.

A good leader could be seen as one who considers their role to be that of liaison with the final say-so, a person who takes all options, considers them and after ruling many out puts the best of them all in to practice. After all the word decision is derived from the Latin word '*decisio*' which comes from the verb '*to cut from*'!

Definitions

Decision-making is a cognitive thought process which selects the most logical choice from a number of given options. When making a decision, a good leader must balance the positives against the negatives of all options and realistically exclude the alternatives. In order to be effective, the ability to forecast the outcome of each option is essential. A good decision can be defined as a course of action (or actions) which are purposely chosen from a set of alternatives to achieve set objectives or outcomes in patient care. Trewatha and Newport (1982) defined the decision-making process as the selection of a course of action from among two or more possibilities in order to arrive at a solution for a given problem. The balance of positives against negatives has to be judged with all the alternatives considered fully and objectively. A paramedic must be able to make the aforementioned forecasts based on knowledge and experience in order to fully envisage the potential outcomes of the decisions that they make. It is being able to put all of these defined components together that enables high standards and low risk of error. Decision-making can also be defined as being an individual's position, opinion or judgement which they have reached following consideration of all the given circumstances. This consideration will enable the paramedic to choose well between numerous courses of action which are available to them using the various cognitive processes: memory, thinking, evaluation, etc. The process of visualizing the likely consequences of the decisions made and the estimation of the importance of the individual factors, concluded by making a choice of the best course of action to take are also an essential part of the decision's success. Defining the external influences on this *best course* can be important too. Influence can be defined as coming from the perception of others, the organization being represented and the environment.

None of the definitions so far have included the untaught or tacit methods by which some leaders make decisions. Many make decisions (clinical or managerial) based on *other* relatively unquantifiable principles. Ask yourself some questions:

- Have you ever had 'just a feeling in your bones' about something?
- Has 'gut instinct' ever played a part in your decision?
- Have you ever heard someone say that they 'just knew something was wrong'?

What are these things all about? Where is the objectivity? How do high-level psychological activity, the use of judgement and the balancing of options and alternatives play a part here? Do all of the other alternative options get truly excluded with these principles and various others? A good decision-maker has a worry that they don't make decisions based on a whim.

Self-evaluation exercise

Have you ever experienced decisions based on a whim? Use the following headings to help you plan your decision-making or reflect upon some decisions you have made in the past.

Decision	Rationale	Outcome

It can be accepted that individual preference and personal values do play a large part in the *weighing up* of options available to paramedics and the final decisions they make. The need for a decision in the first place implies that alternative and equally attractive choices must be considered (Zeleney 1982), and in all circumstances the paramedic will want not only to identify as many of these as possible, but also to choose the option that best fits with not only their professional goals but also their personal desires and values. They will also want the option that appears to have the highest probability of effectiveness in terms of patient care, even when the alternatives have rendered the decision difficult. It is understood that, in general, decision-making is defined as a process of *reducing* uncertainty or doubt regarding alternatives, in order to allow the right (or most right) choice to be selected from among them. Nevertheless, this particular definition places an element of stress on the information-gathering component of the whole decision-making process. Note at this time, however, that uncertainty and doubt are merely reduced, as opposed to completely eliminated. Very few decisions are made by paramedics that offer absolute certainty. This is due to *complete* knowledge about *all* alternatives very rarely being available to them when it is needed. Every decision that a paramedic makes includes a proportion of risk. For sure, this is a difficult concept to accept but is a balancing act.

> You may be willing to take risks. However, whatever risks you take with regard to patient care, you must be prepared to be accountable for the decisions that you make.
>
> (Aston et al. 2010: 125)

If there is a distinct lack of uncertainty about the options available, then this may mean that no decision is really needed. At some stage you will likely see paramedics who thrive upon this lack of choice while continuing to be classed as strong decision-makers! Keep your eyes open for them. Fortunately, there are usually some real-time alternatives available in paramedic practice to choose from. These are not merely pure *do it* or *don't do it* options as these do not really qualify as a true set of alternatives. The options of *do one thing* or *do something else* are more likely to be a realistic and familiar proposition faced daily.

By definition, every clinical or leadership decision has to be made in light of set clinical standards in order to ensure the best use of knowledge, skill and professionalism of judgement. Many of the values, preferences and choices discussed so far are influenced heavily by organizational policies, protocols and guidelines, and quite rightly so. Be aware though that when choosing between two or more options that regional culture, belief and practice will also have played a large part and had some influence in the leader's final decision.

Link to Chapter 4 to read more about organization culture.

Theories of problem solving

The many theories of problem solving and decision-making go hand in hand. As a phase of making a decision, solving a problem is seen as the initial analysis of a difficult situation. The theories of problem solving are overarched by information processing and the identification of specific sub-goals followed by the use of appropriate methods to satisfy those sub-goals. Psychologists have conducted research on problem solving and emphasized the importance of clinicians having an understanding of the full structure of any given problem. Hek and Moule (2006) offered five stages of problem solving and it is only by reading between the lines that the reader can identify where decisions are made (see Box 7.1).

Although the five stages in Box 7.1 are an adaptation of Hek and Moule's (2006) process, it does make them more applicable to paramedics in many given circumstances. Further to this, sometimes the simplest solution comes from a fresh perspective and it is this that encourages high quality decisions to be made while empowering those around. Similar processes can be considered to be of benefit during times of dynamic need. Times when there is dissatisfaction with a situation and problem solving allows the leader to assess, plan and implement a remedy (Standing 2011). Authors have historically presented theories of problem solving that involve a number of aspects – examples such as resources, heuristics, controls and beliefs. Although this style of framework is seen as fairly well developed for mathematical problem solving, it appears to be generally applicable in healthcare too. The ability to problem solve appears to be related to other aspects of cognition including schema, which is the ability to remember similar problems solved in the past and pattern recognition of familiar elements and creativity – the ability to develop new solutions.

Problem-solving skills are fundamental to paramedics and their leaders, but also general medicine and other allied health professions. Problem solving and its underlying theories sit firmly in the world of psychology – it is seen as being the key to leaders reaching a desired objective and moving away from the position that they are currently (and metaphorically) in. In order

---

Box 7.1   The five stages of problem solving

1. Identify the problem.
2. Identify a number of solutions.
3. Evaluate the viability of all options.
4. Select and apply the best option.
5. Evaluate your actions.

Source: Adapted from Hek and Moule (2006).

for paramedics to fully achieve this objective, it is suggested that other elements will need full consideration. These other elements include problem finding and problem shaping – in order to solve the problem, the clinician needs to identify and fully analyse it in the first instance.

And so, in order to understand the way in which we problem solve, we have to consider the way in which we reach that position. It is done through a scientific cognitive process, a process which is structured and includes multiple elements. Elements such as information gathering and processing, environmental consideration, assessment of levels of predictability, intelligence use, memory development and knowledge recall skills.

Some types of problem solving theory

A number of named theories which can lead to a decision's success are suggested:

- *Independent theory* is seen as the construction of particular mind-sets which accomplish specific tasks. This theory can lead to decisions to be made by an individual but only in a single task situation. This particular theory relates to individuals, and, as a result of this, it is not a requirement to get the group perspectives or even consensus from all involved.

- *Content theory* is, as it states, content specific. It considers the manipulation of knowledge regarding a situation to a position where the description is fully analysed and consequently transferred to an outcome process for the final action to be taken.

- *Dynamic theory* is information processing at its sharpest point, and it is suggested as most related to paramedic practice. This type of theory considers multiple changes in behaviour, and attempts to characterize each change and make adaptations immediately in readiness for the next phase of the given situation. This particular theory relies upon memory and peripheral experiences, as opposed to pre-planned, pre-learned or pre-defined processes. The decisions made tend to relate to subtle changes within individual components of the situation at given moments in time. This dynamic theory allows fuller exploration of situations where high risk is present if nothing changes and allows the leader to explore stagnant behaviour.

- *Environmental theory* is perceived as non-experimental. Many changes occur during a single problem-solving situation and this theory suggests that *trying things* is rarely useful. As a preference, a leader should deem it essential to gather ample information about each element of the problem in order to fully identify what information is available and decide how they should go about processing it.

- *Non-statistical theory* can be beneficial to paramedics who may find it difficult to test or assess dynamic, history-dependent pieces of information. In this theory, background information and multiple sources of data are compared and (eventually) attempts are made to measure and consider all the comparisons on offer.

This overview of the theories of problem solving should lead the paramedic towards making positive decisions with positive outcomes. As stated, in order to do this, there needs to be full identification and management of a specific problem towards a satisfactory solution – only positive decision-making will create true instigation of this solution though.

Theories and styles of decision-making

There are many theories of decision-making. These theories may be led by the paramedic's initial motivation to make the decision in the first instance, through to the way in which they may think at the point of decision-making, and finally concluding with them actually making the final decision a reality.

Cognitive dissonance

The initial motivation to make a decision can include a theory of *cognitive dissonance*. Basically, as paramedics (or just as humans), we all want to reduce the potential discomfort of disagreement with others. Simultaneously we have to accept that some of the decisions that we make will lack full consensus or alternatively be perceived as negative by some. There is also a theory which is themed around consistency. Paramedics will always go some way to seeking the comfort of a form of internal alignment as one of the most important elements in decision-making. In addition to feeling empowered, internal alignment allows a leader to feel connected with their inner beliefs and working with their personal values. Initially, this can sound abstract but if we break down what it means to make decisions and then attach values, we can see the benefits.

Self-reflective exercise

Ask yourself some questions:
- Which part of your body makes decisions (heart, head or gut)?
- Does your personality influence the decisions you make?
- Do you have to hold back elements of your personality when making decisions?
- What are the most important values that you apply when decision-making?
- What influences (internal or external) can sway your decision?

Theory of commitment

During the decision-making process, many paramedics will use a theory of commitment. There is a sense of professional and moral obligation in many fields of expertise (paramedicine being just one) to complete a range of actions to a set or defined standard. This theory of commitment is one which many doubt or even neglect at times of strain on resources. But it still remains in existence though affected by what is termed the certainty effect – you need to consider a time when certainty becomes less likely, it's going to have a strong final impact in the situation and therefore the decision(s) that you make.

Bias theory

There is also a theory of bias. A personal or supportive bias which means that the distortion of situational memories goes some way to making bad decisions appear to be good ones, even during the reflective process. This theory can be balanced however, applying confirmation bias during a reflective cycle means that paramedics can seek confirmation that a good decision was made with much better levels of objectivity. But it has to be embedded in reflection deliberately, it cannot occur as part of the process as if by accident.

Theory of motivation

Paramedic motivation to make a decision can also be about not losing face in front of others when they have committed to a specific chain of actions. This is a risky motivator as many circumstances dealt with by paramedics require decisions to be made that should be dynamic and do require multiple inputs at multiple stages. But they are motivation nonetheless. A final motivation can be the want of something that others don't have or have never attempted – an even riskier principle, as it is not driven by knowledge, information and experience in unity, but through an alternative desire!

Link to Chapter 6, team working in paramedic practice.

Ambiguity

During the psychological process of decision-making, a further set of theories play a part. First, it is natural for leaders to consider ambiguity. It is much more preferable to know what may occur than to be completely ignorant. It is commonly understood that a decision based on ignorance has a high chance of failure. Recognizing personal and professional biases and ensuring that we reduce the risk of information bias are also keys (Croskerry 2002). There is the chance that we may not compensate fully for biases that we have but recognizing this as a concept is certainly a start.

Heuristic-systematic persuasion

Situational circumstances mean that paramedics have become highly skilled at using shortcuts and logic to interpret the numerous arguments that they are presented with. This is known as the heuristic-systematic persuasion model. Heuristic means that the decision made is experience based and allows a higher degree of problem solving, development and discovery to be engaged in. Where a widened search is not perceived as being practical by a leader, heuristic methods can be engaged in to accelerate the process of coming to a satisfactory decision. These are mental shortcuts which are used to ease the cognitive load of making a decision. Examples of this method include such traditional terminology as using a *general rule*, an *educated guess*, an *intuitive judgement* or *common sense*.

Reflection: points to consider

- Think about a patient case where it has taken longer to establish a potential diagnosis, due to the clinicians taking shortcuts and making assumptions, based on previous experiences. During this time, vital information may have been overlooked or discarded because of the paramedic working on a heuristic.
- With the benefit of reflection, can you now see what was overlooked and the danger that heuristics presents? Remember, no two patients are the same, even if superficially their presentation of illness may seem very similar.

Hyperbolic discounting

In such dynamic circumstances such as those in which paramedics function, hyperbolic discounting is a philosophy which plays a large part. Paramedics are in a profession which demonstrates a preference for a decision that gives visible outcomes sooner rather than later. Many paramedics consider discounting the true value of later reward, demonstrating preference for short-term benefits. Hyperbolic discounting as a decision-making style refers directly to the tendency of people to choose a *smaller-sooner* reward over a *larger-later* reward, a style which fits the needs of much of the care that paramedics deliver. Many clinicians will work to this style but it is seen by others in this contemporary and changing profession as a potential defect of human reasoning, an irrational bias considered to be a temporal myopia (Worthy et al. 2012). Not unlike visual myopia, temporal myopia creates a decrease of clarity with distance, but instead of the sense of sight being affected, it is the sense of perception. Instead of instigating a cautious approach, the paramedic's response has the potential to be reduced in terms of the importance of the longer-term outcomes for their patient. Subsequent consequences occurring later in a patient's recovery, whether they are good or bad, are at risk of having a lot less bearing on decisions the further they are in the future, and this could be the case even when life is at stake.

Analytical decision-making models

A further theory involves information processing, a theory deeply rooted in medical decision-making. It is a model which uses a deductive approach to assist logical reasoning, an approach which sits very comfortably with many paramedics. Many healthcare professionals have adopted this information processing approach to help them with their clinical decision-making. Analytical decision-making models, such as this, have been used to assist in diagnostic reasoning, a process key to making decisions in the pre- and out-of-hospital setting. These models make the assumption that the decision-maker's thought processes are going to follow logical routes which have the potential to be analysed until a clear decision has been made.

It is during the process of making key decisions that specific clinical experiences become so important to this particular analytical model. A study by Hedberg and Sätterlund Larsson (2003) demonstrated the ability of nurses to think ahead of situations and then adopt preventative strategies to circumstances. This process is connected with the use of intervention-based decisions and potential adverse events, but it also encouraged those nurses to act independently. It is commensurate with the rationalized, analytical and deductive models of clinical decision-making used regularly but not necessarily recognized by paramedics. This model of decision-making does have its drawbacks. Hypotheses regarding outcomes may be incorrect and this could lead to the development of propositions which are essentially wrong. This approach to decision-making offers the assumption that knowledge is available and information is accurate. In real life, though, many of the decisions made by paramedics possess a high degree of uncertainty, meaning that more advanced thought has to be offered to the benefit of any decision but the same degree of thought has to be offered to its alternative potential consequences too.

Unconscious thought theory

There are times when the paramedic can use tacit decision-making and this is perceived as unconscious thought theory, a situation where we allow our subconscious to do the thinking. Many attributes of unconscious thought theory are taken from research on the various forms of psychology. Together these forms of psychology can portray abilities way beyond those of conscious thought. Unconscious thought is reminiscent of some of the classical views that emerged so many years ago. The term *bias correction* has been banded about by many authors. The concept to which this expression relates is a risk for all paramedics. We all have biases, these are largely dependent on our own experiences and set of beliefs, which lead to us making judgements and forming stereotypes. As professionals, we act in a manner befitting our professional body and take pride in the anti-discriminatory, high standard of care that we provide. If we are self-aware, we know and understand our own biases. As well-meaning professionals in difficult circumstances, the paramedic may unconsciously over-compensate for their bias when caring for some patients. For example, a paramedic may have an adult with Down's Syndrome in their family. The paramedic may find themselves employing strategies that they would use in their own family, if they attend a family with a Down's Syndrome child requiring care. This may involve being over-familiar with the family, telling them that you understand, what your colleagues may describe as being 'over the top'. In the reverse, the paramedic may find that this type of call is too personal and raises emotions that they cannot manage in a work environment, consequently, they may distance themselves from the situation, appearing detached and unfriendly. This is a personal example, but bias correction can also occur in response to a policy directive or peer pressure.

Reflection: points to consider

Have you ever offered care beyond that required by the specific patient, either as a result of policy, peer pressure or your own biases?

It is this type of example which should be considered cautiously, the decision that is being made about patient care and scene management should always be based upon the circumstances and information offered and not on the desire to go beyond the needs and requirements of the time. There is a need for comparisons to be made, comparisons to previous experiences, whether actual, perceived or simulated, first- or second-hand. This perceptual contrast will go some way to effecting positive decisions to be made based on historical levels of success and failure. During the education of the paramedic (traditional ambulance-based or contemporary higher education orientated), it has always been, and remains important to prime learners in order to set up memories for the future. This priming includes the use of valuable experiences such as:

- situational theory/case examples
- role play
- simulation
- third party observation.

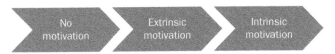

Figure 7.2   The professional motivation continuum.

Self-determination and self-regulation

The final theoretical considerations to make in an autonomous profession are those of self-determination and self-regulation. In equal measures, these theories alone can ensure that the paramedic is motivated to a high standard while simultaneously able to control their emotions, feelings and urges. Self-determination theory aims to go some way to explaining goal-centred behaviours. Professional motivation lives on a continuum (see Figure 7.2), with no motivation at all on the left, extrinsic at the centre and intrinsic on the right.

Extrinsic motivation is driven by external influences. It is a less preferred state but far better than none at all, a complete absence of motivation which has the potential to lead to minimal (if any) decision-making occurring at all. Intrinsic motivation is seen as being the ideal, whereupon paramedics engage in decision-making activities due to internal factors and these activities are perceived as most likely to be made for the right personal and professional reasons.

One critical component of all of these theories concerns the depth to which the clinician is able to meet their own basic psychological needs. The more they are able to achieve these basic psychological needs, the more likely it will be that their behaviour is truly self-determined and deliverable. On the other hand, self-regulation describes the full control and management of clinical performance by means of a number of processes. These processes include:

• maintaining behaviour which is focused on outcome;

• defining strategies for overall achievement;

• alteration of behaviours or strategies in order to optimize performance.

In summary, as Figure 7.3 demonstrates, the key to sound clinical decision-making is dependent on three key areas: knowledge, experience and the information available.

If any of the key factors are lacking, this will affect the quality of the clinical decision. It is the paramedic's responsibility to ensure thorough assessment is completed to obtain all the information required. To use their experience, but be careful not to rely on heuristics (using a previous case and expecting this patient's case to be exactly the same, thus potentially missing valuable cues and clues to the differences). Applying their knowledge to the given

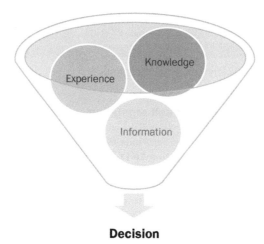

Decision

Figure 7.3 The key factors required to make clinical decisions.

situation and exploring other options, reasons and causes, ensuring the best clinical decision is made for their patient.

Conclusion

This chapter has allowed the consideration of the paramedic's ability to make decisions as a leader. A good leader has to be in a position to make decisions on behalf of not only themselves but also those who are either in their charge or of less experience or grade. Nevertheless, it is important to note that not all leaders hold superior positions, some leaders lead from within. Although there may be managers, officers, supervisors, mentors and preceptors developed or promoted in to their position, true leaders can and do exist naturally.

The main focus of this chapter has been on the subject of decision-making as a broad concept and within that concept are such topics as problem solving and the understanding of basic psychology and theories. Decision-making is wrongly perceived as being a simple and tacit (unspoken) activity, but it takes a combination of knowledge of the subject, experience of the circumstances and information about the situation to make the best decision.

This combination with an input of confident and competent leadership develops the potential for a higher standard of clinical or managerial decision to be made. The chapter has looked at some definitions of terms used in decision-making for the purpose of clarification and further discussion or debate and further to this, a number of theories of historical perspectives have been considered and offered for you to make comparisons.

Chapter key points

- To be a good paramedic leader you have to make good decisions.
- Experience, knowledge and information are key requirements for good paramedic decisions.
- Circumstances sometimes dictate that paramedics have limited information.
- Decisive paramedic leaders can shape care delivery at all levels and empower paramedics.
- Decisions are subjective, primarily based on individual position, opinion or judgement.
- Making a decision reduces uncertainty and doubt but does not remove it.
- The ability to problem solve is a prerequisite to decision-making.
- A number of key theories combine in order to problem solve.
- Cognitive dissonance is a human trait which can act as a barrier to decision-making.
- Paramedics have to be cautious using educated guesses, common sense or intuitive judgements.
- Paramedics have traditionally aimed for more short-term benefits, this needs to change in order to deliver more effective care.
- Education can develop knowledge and experience but not information.

References and suggested reading

Aston, L., Wakefield, J. and McGown, R. (eds) (2010) *The Student Nurse Guide to Decision-making in Practice*. Maidenhead: McGraw-Hill.

Croskerry, P. (2002) Achieving quality in clinical decision-making: cognitive strategies and detection of bias, *Academic Emergency Medicine*, 9(11): 1184–204.

Godolphin, W. (2009) Shared decision-making, *Healthcare Quarterly*, 12.

Gurbutt, R. (2011) *Decision-making and Healthcare Management for Frontline Staff*. Oxford: Radcliffe Publishing.

Hedberg, B. and Sätterlund Larrson, J. (2003) Observations, confirmations and strategies: useful tools in decision-making process for nurses in practice? *Journal of Clinical Nursing*, 12(2): 215–22.

Hek, G. and Moule, P. (2006) *Making Sense of Research*, 3rd edn. London: Sage.

NHS Leadership Academy (2012) The NHS Leadership Academy: delivering the strategy. Available at: http://www.leadershipacademy.nhs.uk/.

NHS Leadership Academy (2013) *Healthcare Leadership Model: The Nine Dimensions of Leadership Behaviour*. Version 1.0. Leeds: NHS Leadership Academy. Available at: www.leadershipacademy.nhs.uk/leadershipmodel (accessed 26 November 2013).

Nursing and Midwifery Council (2010) *Standards for Pre-Registration Nursing Education*. London: NMC.

Standing, M. (2011) *Clinical Judgement and Decision-making for Nursing Students.* London: Sage.

St Mary's Healthcare, Amsterdam (online). Available at: http://www.smha.org/about/mission_vision_values.cfm (accessed March 2013).

The Guardian (online). Available at: http://www.guardian.co.uk/healthcare-network/2013/feb/14/francis-report-nhs-leadership (accessed February 2013).

Trewatha, R.L. and Newport, G.M. (1982) *Management,* 3rd edn. London: Business Publication

Worthy, D.A., Otto, A.R. and Maddox, W.T. (2012) Working memory load and temporal myopia in dynamic decision-making, *Journal of Experimental Psychology,* 38(6): 1640–58.

Zeleny, M. (1982) *Multiple Criteria Decision-making.* Maidenhead: McGraw-Hill.

Useful websites

http://www.businessballs.com/problemsolving.htm.

http://www.cliffsnotes.com/study_guide/The-DecisionMaking-Process.topicArticleId-8944,articleId-8863.html.

http://decision-quality.com/intro.php.

http://www.leadershipacademy.nhs.uk/discover/leadership-framework/setting-direction/making-decisions/.

8 Managing and leading change

Surinder Walia

Introduction

The aim of this chapter is to discuss and explore the importance of effectively managing and leading systematic, unprecedented large-scale change in today's ever evolving, complex healthcare systems within the National Health Service (NHS). Components of the Leadership Framework (DH 2011) and the NHS Change Model (2012) will be explored, to enable paramedics, ambulance clinicians, nurse leaders/managers, and allied healthcare professionals to apply these theories to their every-day practice when leading, managing and facilitating transformational change, in promoting excellence in quality of care to all patients and clients across all sectors.

Within the current health service the vision and strategy are to provide cost-effective, high quality, compassionate care for all by ensuring excellent health and well-being outcomes, delivered by a highly empowered workforce, who manage and lead ongoing change effectively across systems of care at both local and national level, uncontrolled by bureaucracy and hierarchy (DH 2009, 2010, 2012; The King's Fund 2011). Within ever evolving and challenging environments, clinical leaders and allied care practitioners such as paramedics and nurses are expected to embrace and sustain change, ensure processes and systems of care are streamlined and promote transformational workplace cultures in readiness for forthcoming changes. It is considered that only then can there be a successful drive forward to new ways of working in which facilitative, transformational organizational and system changes being proposed by government directives and legislation can be aligned.

Leading and managing change is not a new concept or phenomenon in health or healthcare delivery systems, as it could be argued that change has been a continuous constant since the introduction of the NHS in 1948, with practitioners having to adapt and develop to ongoing changes made to their organizations and services by both internal as well as external influences. A clear example of this constant change can be seen within the ambulance service in the last decade, in which the main agenda has been to modernize the service, with the ultimate aim of transforming it into a world class, efficient and streamlined mobile healthcare service for the NHS (DH 2005). However, it is felt by paramedics and healthcare professionals alike that the present changes being advocated, facilitated and implemented within today's healthcare settings are considered to be on a much larger scale and pace with more far-reaching consequences and effects than seen in the past.

In the past, various leadership competency frameworks were introduced to help develop individuals and aid the process of change and change management within the NHS, including the Leadership Qualities Framework (NHS 2002), the Medical Leadership Competency Framework (NHS 2009), the Clinical Leadership Competency Framework (NHS 2011) and more recently the Leadership Framework (LF) (DH 2011) and Healthcare Leadership Model (2013), in which key domains from these previous frameworks are entrenched. These frameworks have been designed and advocated in an effort to assist staff in improving their own personal leadership abilities so that they in turn can drive and lead the necessary changes in a positive, proactive and efficient manner within their healthcare settings. In addition, more recently there has been the introduction of the NHS Change Model (NHS 2012), to assist NHS commissioners and providers to deliver a quality service by using a universally applied model of change, understood and used by all healthcare professionals working within the NHS.

Reflection: points to consider

When you are introducing change in your everyday working practice, how many times have you considered using a structured approach in leading and facilitating this change?

Ask yourself: was *your* way of implementing change successful, or could the process of change be managed differently?

Self-evaluation exercise

Undertake Section 5, 'Setting Direction' of the NHS Leadership Academy's self-assessment activity. It focuses on identifying the contexts for change. This document can be accessed from: http://www.leadershipacademy.nhs.uk/wp-content/uploads/2012/11/NHSLeadership-Framework-CLCFSelfAssessmentTool.pdf.

Leading a team through change

There are various definitions of change, the following are two current examples:

> Change is a process that is driven by forces that motivate a person or an organisation to consider what needs altering.
>
> (Finkleman and Kenner 2013: 252)

> Energy for change is the capacity and drive of a team, organisation or system to act and make the difference necessary to achieve its goals.
>
> (Bevan and Hunt 2013: 6)

When any change is introduced that affects the status quo, this will evoke differing degrees of resistance and anxiety within the workforce. Even though change has been inevitable within the NHS, anecdotal evidence suggests that instead of embracing change, either planned or unplanned staff working in healthcare and healthcare settings have generally viewed any changes imposed on them by a top-down transactional leadership approach with suspicion and scepticism, resulting in resistance and at times non-compliance to the change process. It is felt that at times inexperienced leaders or managers have attempted to initiate complex, organizational change within their working environments without a great deal of success, due to their lack of expertise in leading change.

In twenty-first-century contemporary healthcare environments, intentional transformational change for improvement is driven by both internal and external forces, resulting in either a planned or unplanned change depending on the circumstances. For example, change is constant in primary, secondary and voluntary healthcare sectors, with planned change which can arise as a result of organizational restructuring and changes to infrastructures, while unplanned change can result from unpredictable workforce shortages and poor management. Marquis and Huston (2012) suggest planned change is when the leader/manager intentionally uses their knowledge and skills to instigate change in an organized and cohesive manner, while they state unplanned change occurs as an accidental change or a *change of drift*. Similarly, Barr and Dowding (2012) state that planned change managed purposefully and efficiently by the leader/manager, will ensure healthcare professionals embrace the change positively, however, they maintain that imposed unplanned change can result in negative and uncooperative behaviours exhibited by the workforce, arguably as seen on numerous occasions in today's healthcare settings.

Link to Chapter 4 to read about the potential effect that change has on organizational culture.

Evidence shows that the importance of having skilled healthcare professionals and a motivated workforce, led by personnel who have the managerial and leadership abilities in which to effectively lead and facilitate continuous change using a transformational approach, has been widely recognized as being an integral part of an effective leadership role. Given the continual pressures experienced by healthcare professionals on a daily and at times on an hourly basis, resulting from a constant state of change, both planned and unplanned within their everyday practice, it is paramount that the change process is led and managed by experienced leaders/managers.

Reflection: points to consider
- When did you last initiate a change within your working environment?
- Was it a planned or unplanned change?
- Ask yourself, why do planned changes work more efficiently?
- Do you manage unplanned changes well? If not, why not?

Leadership style of the change agent

Burton and Ormrod (2011) maintain that 'not all leaders are managers', but they argue that 'all managers need to be leaders'. It is based on this premise that for the remainder of this chapter the paramedic leader/manager will be discussed as an interchangeable role and will be referred to as the change agent. Marquis and Huston (2012: 163) define a change agent as 'A person skilled in the theory and implementation of planned change, to deal appropriately with these very real human emotions and to connect and balance all aspects of the organisation that will be affected by that change.' This implies that an ad hoc approach in managing the change process is not considered sufficient, but care and thought need to be given in ensuring the right person is deployed to drive forward the change required if success of the planned change is sought.

Transformational and transactional styles

A shared vision is the catalyst that drives transformational organizational change, so the effectiveness and the success of this change are greatly dependent on the leadership/management abilities of the change agent. Whatever the driving force for the need to make a change, it affects the equilibrium and stability within an organization either in a positive or negative fashion, depending on the expertise of the change agent promoting the change. Cultures within organizations dictate leadership behaviours. A transformational culture will mean the change agent is nurtured to lead within a supportive and empowered environment, the experience being positive. This is in direct opposition to the transactional culture of an organization, where the change agent's experience is likely to be viewed as rather negative. In spite of this, the expectation and belief remain that the appointed change agent will be instrumental in effectively initiating and facilitating adaptation to changes made within their workplace, using a proactive and proficient change management process. In reality, this is not always the case as evidence suggests that not all change agents have the necessary theoretical knowledge of how to competently manage the change process, are not capable of managing the changed equilibrium, and do not have the necessary skills or characteristics to act as an effective change agent within their working environments.

It is apparent from the empirical literature, vast research and by the introduction of directives such as the NHS Change Model and Leadership Framework that there is a clear move and drive to changing, strengthening and building leadership approaches used within healthcare settings. There is definite emphasis on leaders and managers promoting and facilitating the necessary changes taking place within the current changing healthcare systems by embracing change and promoting positive working environments. There is a move away from the previously traditional leadership style (see Box 8.1) which predominately focused upon using a transactional,

---

Box 8.1   Transactional leaders – the *top-down* approach

- Autocratic
- Hierarchical
- Matriarchal
- Focus on individual gain
- Reactive
- Little or no autonomy for staff
- Extensive power and control
- Concerned with accomplishing tasks rather than worrying about relationships
- Given power to reward or punish team performance

Box 8.2 Transformational leaders – the *bottom-up* approach

- Charismatic
- Highly visible/flexible
- Committed to the organization's vision or ideal
- Inspirational and autonomous motivator
- Intellectually stimulated
- Self-aware/self-efficient
- Encourages culture of creativity and critical thinking
- Questions status quo
- Empowers others
- People orientated
- Leads collaboratively, using a cascading or chain reaction effect
- Proactive
- Emphasis on personal ability/skill
- Promotes employee development

---

hierarchical and autocratic approach to leadership (Alimo-Metcalfe and Alban-Metcalfe 2002; Thyer 2003; Burns 2003; Murphy 2005), in which, according to Doody and Doody (2012), staff were over-managed, lacked autonomy and were restricted in the decision- and change-making process.

The favoured move is currently towards a more transformational paradigm (see Box 8.2) which promotes individual empowerment, recognizes and values the expertise where leadership behaviours are described as being effective change agents and is deemed to be crucial in the present, ever changing healthcare leadership (Finkelman 2012; Health Foundation 2011; Sorensen et al. 2008; Burns 2003; Bass and Avolio 1994; Conger and Kanungo 1987). In the transformational leadership approach the change agent can be any healthcare professional such as a student paramedic (as exemplified in case study 8.1), a paramedic, a Specialist paramedic, an Advanced paramedic or a Consultant paramedic to name but a few, regardless of their hierarchical position within their organization.

Importantly, the individual who takes on the role of change agent needs to be an innovative and creative risk taker who has the personal skills and leadership characteristics to communicate positively the shared vision, to engage, motivate and gain commitment of their teams in order to facilitate and implement changes to healthcare delivery systems, so that the vision can then become a reality. Finkelman (2012) supports this view when she advocates that the change agent will only be considered effective in the change management process, if the leader exhibits charisma, has enabling abilities, is instrumental in providing necessary resources

---

Case study 8.1

In many higher education institutions (HEIs), final year students undertake modules where leadership and managing change are explored, covering many aspects discussed in this text. As part of the students' assessment, they may be asked to plan a small-scale change in the practice area. This will involve exploring the leadership style of the staff in their placement area, group dynamics and using a managing change model to crystallize their thoughts and plan how best to implement the change. Students are often encouraged to read about many change models and choose one, explaining the rationale for their choice.

In clinical areas where staff are well informed about the curriculum of their local HEI students have been asked to actually implement their ideas. This starts with a pilot in one or two stations, evaluating the change process and potentially *rolling out* to a larger area. The success of this approach relies on the fact that the change is small-scale, not reliant on money being forthcoming, but aids practice staff, for example, a laminated sheet of common Makaton signs.

This can be a win-win situation, with students feeling empowered, able to put their plans into practice and experiencing the potential pitfalls of leading a change in a real clinical practice environment. They are starting their leadership careers. For clinical staff, they are able to support leadership from within the organization, develop new practice ideas and nurture the paramedics of the future. All of this process benefits the patient in the long term, directly or indirectly.

---

and is a missionary agent who communicates effectively the organizational vision to their staff.

It is important to note at this stage, that though the chosen and preferred style of leadership in government directives and legislation seems to be the transformational leadership approach, some theorists consider that the use of this approach alone will hinder and be insufficient for the excessive level of change and development required within the present healthcare settings, and they maintain that certain transactional characteristics should also be deployed if greater success is to be achieved. For example, Doody and Doody (2012) give caution to the use of transformational leadership alone as they argue that the change agent exposes themselves as well as their organizations to high levels of risk, if other leaders/managers at a greater hierarchal level are not able to intervene using a transactional approach when needed to prevent errors and mistakes being made by the acting change agent.

The overall consensus within the literature promotes leadership characteristics and attributes to be utilized from both transactional and transformational leadership styles, if the necessary change is to be effectively promoted and change management policies are to be successfully facilitated and implemented by the change agent (Bass 1985, 1994; Alimo-Metcalfe and Alban-Metcalfe 2002; Millward and Bryan 2005; Marquis and Huston 2012).

As a leader, you have the power to influence, and you make a choice to either influence negatively or positively.

(Gitomer 2011: 1)

Self-evaluation exercise
- Do you consider yourself to be a change agent?
- Are you a risk taker?
- List the personal qualities and skills that *you* consider you already have as a positive change agent.
- Now ask your line manager and your team to also make a list of personal attributes/skills they feel you exhibit, then compare the two lists against Box 8.1 and Box 8.2.

Self-evaluation exercise

Undertake Section 1 of the NHS Leadership Academy's personal qualities activity. This can be found at: http://www.leadershipacademy.nhs.uk/wp-content/uploads/2012/11/NHSLeadership-Framework-CLCFSelfAssessmentTool.pdf.

Leadership competency frameworks

The use of leadership competency frameworks and interactive leadership theories which address the leader/follower relationship have continued to evolve over the last few years, in an attempt to improve individual clinical leadership skills and abilities so that the needs of the rapidly changing competitive, market-driven and person-focused environments can be satisfied. For example, the emergence of the Emotional Intelligence (EI) theory by Goleman (1998), in which the focus remains on the leader, who has in-depth insight and understanding about one's own emotional self-awareness, self-management, self-motivation, self-empathy and social awareness and understands its direct and indirect impact on the emotions of others. Goleman maintains that a manager's emotional intelligence can have a powerful, positive effect on how well the organization performs and he argues that without emotional intelligence, a manager cannot be an effective leader. Leaders need to remember:

Your people are a direct reflection of you. They watch you. They follow you. They measure you. They listen to you. If you want them to be dedicated to you, you have to be dedicated to them.

(Gitomer 2011: 27)

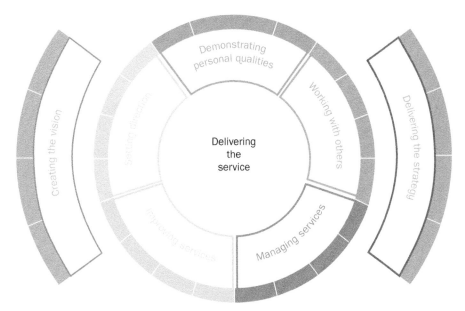

Figure 8.1   The Clinical Leadership Competency Framework. *Source*: NHS Leadership Academy (2011a).

The NHS has published the Leadership Framework and the Clinical Leadership Competency Framework which have been introduced to be used by all healthcare professionals (Leadership Academy 2011a 2011b), irrespective of their clinical role or position within the organization (see Figure 8.1). It has been created and built around existing leadership frameworks, in a wish that all personnel working within healthcare settings aspire and work towards shared values and ideals. This framework is a free, web-based developmental tool designed to improve personal leadership abilities of all healthcare professionals working within the NHS as it is considered that all staff have a shared responsibility for the success or failure of the organization in which they work. The clinical staff overseeing the students' change project in case study 8.1 could introduce the Leadership Framework to the student, further developing their understanding and appreciation of available tools.

This tool is intended to be used as a benchmarking aid along with other career or skill-based developmental tools such as the NHS Change Model (Figure 8.2), which assists in improving personal leadership qualities and skills and promoting effective change. The Leadership Framework is designed to help individuals identify and understand what stage they are at within their own leadership progression and their leadership development, by benchmarking their progress against the relevant domains based upon their respective level of leadership (see Box 8.3 and Box 8.4) and four key stages (see Box 8.5) within this structure.

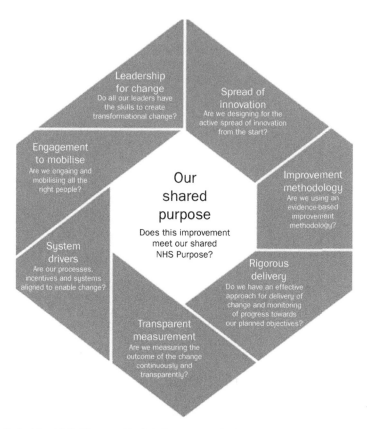

Figure 8.2 The NHS Change Model. *Source*: NHS (2012).

Reflection: points to consider

- Think about your annual meeting with your manager (individual performance review, individual development review – there are numerous names for this process).
- Are the NHS Leadership Framework or NHS Change Model used as part of the process?
- Have you ever been directed to the Leadership Academy's website for the online self-assessment tools (that have been referred to throughout this book)?

Once this awareness and level of ability have been established, the individual can then work towards improving and strengthening their personal leadership characteristics, behaviours and knowledge, with the aim of becoming competent leaders and change agents who promote a high quality service.

Box 8.3   Five core domains (1–5)

Demonstrating Personal Qualities

Working with others

Managing services

Improving services

Setting direction

Source: Leadership Academy (2011a).

Additionally two further domains, 6 and 7 core domains (see Box 8.4), have been devised to provide specific guidance for those who are in (or are aspiring to) the most senior positions of leadership within the profession or organization. However, this does not mean that others cannot assist in the organization achieving these, or aspire or thrive towards achieving these domains.

Box 8.4   Domains 6 and 7

- Domain 6 – Creating the Vision: Effective leadership involves creating a compelling vision for the future, and communicating this within and across organizations.
- Domain 7 – Delivering the Strategy: Effective leadership involves delivering the strategy by developing and agreeing strategic plans that place patient care at the heart of the service, and ensuring that these are translated into achievable operational plans.

Reflection: points to consider

- How much do you know about the Leadership Framework?
- Do you know which one of the four stages you are currently leading at?

Self- reflective exercise

Now work through the remaining elements 2, 3 and 4 of the NHS Leadership Academy's personal qualities activity. This can be found at: http:// www.leadershipacademy.nhs.uk/wp-content/uploads/2012/11/NHSLeadership-Framework-CLCFSelfAssessmentTool.pdf.

Have you identified any areas which need developing?

Box 8.5   Four key stages

Low risk, leadership impact on own practice and immediate team only.

More risk involved, leadership impact on whole service and across other teams.

Far-reaching risk, leadership impact across other departments/disciplines and within the wider organization.

High risk involvement, leadership across whole networks both internally and externally, at national and international levels to support healthcare systems.

Change models

The introduction and use of change models and change theories to assist in the change management process by a change agent are not new concepts or phenomena. There is a plethora of literature which discusses various change models and adaptive versions of original models to be found (see Box 8.6 for one of the key seminal models by Lewin, used and adapted over time and which will be one of two change models discussed in this chapter). As highlighted in case study 8.1, numerous change models are available, but Lewin and the NHS Change Model are a good place to begin your reading and understanding.

Lewin's change model

Importantly, during the moving phase of Lewin's change model, the change agent needs to ensure that the driving forces (drivers that facilitate and aid

---

Box 8.6   Lewin's force-field model of change: three key stages

Unfreezing: The team understands the need to change; the change agent gains the enthusiasm and motivation of these individuals by taking into consideration the culture of the environment, the psychological and physical impact the desired change may have on the workforce.

Moving: Planned change occurs, in which the change agent identifies, drives and implements strategies to initiate the planned journey of change.

Refreezing: Stabilization of the change; over time, the change agent re-adjusts aspects of the working environment so that the status quo can once again be restored, once the change process has been implemented and distinguished.

(Lewin 1951)

change) always surpass any possible restraining forces (barriers which impede or prevent change), if compliance and a positive approach to the planned change are sought and administered (Marquis and Huston 2012). For example, in healthcare and healthcare environments, in the unfreezing phase, the change agents must first of all decide whether the change to the existing systems is indeed necessary, then seek full consent and cooperation from the workforce so that any new legislation and government directive can be instigated and aligned, according to the new ways of working in the attempt to radically reform the NHS. It is without a shadow of a doubt that change agents working within the present NHS will be required to make unprecedented and challenging changes within their working environments if the desired quality and financial initiatives and outcomes are to be achieved. With the introduction of General Practitioner (GP) consortia and commissioning bodies, change is inevitable; however, the fundamental characteristic is how the required change is driven forward among the existing workforce.

The NHS Change Model

The NHS Change Model (seen in Figure 8.2) is the current change model introduced to health and healthcare professionals to deal with the ongoing demands and challenges of the ever changing face of the NHS and to help drive transformational change at a large scale across all sectors and disciplines within the NHS.

As can be seen in Figure 8.2 this model consists of eight components:

1. Our shared purpose

2. Engagement to mobilize

3. Leadership for change

4. Improvement methodology

5. Rigorous delivery

6. Transparent measurement

7. System drivers

8. Spread of innovation.

This model has been devised and formulated by utilizing and building upon existing experience, expertise and improvement knowledge of previously used change models and change theories used in health environments. It uses a simplistic, common language understood by all healthcare professionals. Although in this chapter the focus has been on the 'Leadership for change' component of this model, it is important to recognize that all eight parts of the model are necessary for a successful change transformation. Therefore, all parts of the model should be used interchangeably and not separated to avoid an over-reliance on any one component. For the Leadership for change component, it is stated that through shared leadership and collaborative working, the large-scale change needed within the NHS can be successfully implemented by all healthcare professionals, regardless of their hierarchal position within their organizations. These change agents need to act as inspirational role models and have the necessary facilitative leadership qualities, knowledge and skills to create, support and drive trans-formational change successfully, using all eight components of the change model. This model holds the belief that when discussing or leading change, this implies that change 'is connected to a purpose and that people are con-nected to the change in a very open way' (NHS Change Model 2012: 2). This suggests imposed change should be avoided and that planned, informed compliance will drive the necessary large-scale change more successfully. This view clearly reflects and reinforces the findings and discussion at the beginning of this chapter.

Link to Chapter 6 for discussion on team roles.

Reflection: points to consider

- What do you actually know about change models?
- Are you aware of Lewin's change model and how to use it in your everyday practice?
- Are you able to facilitate all eight components of the NHS Change Model equally and interchangeably, when initiating or driving change within the workplace?
- As a change agent, which aspects of the two models above do you need to develop?

Conclusion

Hopefully, this chapter has provided you with a brief overview of the impor-tance of using recognized strategies and competency-based frameworks when managing and leading both planned and unplanned change within your clinical practice and organization. Continuous transformational change within healthcare environments is inevitable in the foreseeable future, so it is paramount that all healthcare practitioners realize this and embrace this fact rather than shy away from it, so that unimpeded change can occur as required. The need to incorporate aspects of change willingly within every-day practice is inescapable and unavoidable.

However, the importance of managing any change process efficiently by an able and qualified change agent cannot be over-emphasized, whether it is at strategic, service or at frontline level. That clinicians and practitioners need to have a keen awareness of their own clinical leadership abilities and skills cannot be stressed too strongly. They are required to manage ongoing change within their complex working environments, so they need to ensure they are equipped to lead this process with confidence and competence. Only when the change process is sufficiently embraced and managed effectively by all healthcare professionals, can the planned reforms of the NHS be truly fulfilled, in which the ultimate aim is to provide universal high quality care for all.

Chapter key points

- In today's twenty-first-century health and healthcare systems, change remains a constant which needs to be managed effectively.

- If excellence in health care and healthcare systems is to be achieved, change needs to be led effectively.

- Within any leadership role, individuals need to understand the required leadership expectation of their role.

- Individuals need to be aware of their own leadership style when acting as a change agent.

- Individuals need to be aware of the self-help tools available from the NHS and use them to enhance their own professional development and leadership expertise.

- Awareness of change models should improve the clinician's understanding of change, provide a clear structured way to think about implementing any change – hopefully improving the chances of change success.

- A wide variety of strategies and competency-based leadership models have been introduced that practitioners and clinicians can use when managing and leading the process of change.

References and suggested reading

Alimo-Metcalfe, B. and Alban-Metcalfe, J. (2002) The great and the good, *People Management*, 10: 32–4.

Darr, J. and Dowding, L. (2012) *Leadership in Health Care*, 2nd edn. London: Sage.

Bass, B.M. (1985) *Leadership and Performance Beyond Expectations*. New York: Free Press.

Bass, B.M. and Avolio, B.J. (eds) (1994) *Improving Organisational Effectiveness Through Transformational Leadership*. Thousand Oaks, CA: Sage.

Bevan, H. and Hunt, R. (2013) *Building and Aligning Energy for Change: A Review of Published and Grey Literature, Initial Concept Testing and Development*. York: NHS Landmark Health Economics Consortium.

Burns, J.M. (2003) *Transforming Leadership*. New York: Grove/Atlantic Inc.

Burton, R. and Ormrod, G. (2011) *Nursing: Transition to Professional Practice*. Oxford: Oxford University Press.

Conger, J.A. and Kanungo, R.N. (1987) Toward a behavioural theory of charismatic leadership in organisational settings, *Academy of Management Review*, 12: 637–47.

Department of Health (2002) *NHS Leadership Qualities Framework*. London: Department of Health.

Department of Health (2005) *Taking Healthcare to the Patient: Transforming NHS Ambulance Services.* London: Department of Health.

Department of Health (2009) *Inspiring Leaders: Leadership for Quality.* London: Department of Health.

Department of Health (2010) *Equity and Excellence: Liberating the NHS.* London: Department of Health.

Department of Health (2011) *Leadership Framework.* London: Department of Health.

Department of Health (2012) *Compassion in Practice: Nursing, Midwifery and Care Staff, Our Vision and Strategy.* London: Department of Health.

Doody, O. and Doody, C. (2012) Transformational leadership in nursing practice, *British Journal of Nursing*, 21(20): 1212–18.

Finkelman, A. (2012) *Leadership and Management for Nurses: Core Competencies for Quality Care*, 2nd edn. Harlow: Pearson.

Finkelman, A. and Kenner, C. (2013) *Professional Nursing Concepts: Competencies for Quality Leadership*, 2nd edn. Cambridge, MA: Jones & Bartlett.

Gitomer, J. (2011) *Little Book of Leadership: The 12.5 Strengths of Responsible, Reliable, Remarkable Leaders that Create Results, Rewards and Resilience.* London: John Wiley & Sons.

Goleman, D. (1998) *Working with Emotional Intelligence.* New York: Bantam Books.

Health Foundation (2011) *What's Leadership Got to Do with It?* London: Health Foundation UK.

Lewin, K. (1951) *Field Theory in Social Sciences.* New York: Harper & Row.

Marquis, B. and Huston, C. (2012) *Leadership and Management Tools for the New Nurse: A Case Study Approach.* Philadelphia, PA: Lippincott Williams & Wilkins.

Murphy, L. (2005) Transformational leadership: a cascading chain reaction, *Journal of Nursing Management*, 13: 128–36.

Millward, L.J. and Bryan, K. (2005) Clinical leadership in health care: a position statement, *International Journal of Health Care Assurance*, 18(2/3): R13.

NHS Change Model (2012) Available at: www.changemodel.nhs.uk/pg/dashboard (accessed 13 October 2013).

NHS Institute for Innovation and Improvement (2005) *NHS Leadership Qualities Framework.* Available at: http://www.nhsleadershipqualities.nhs.uk (accessed 27 July 2013).

NHS Institute for Innovation and Improvement (2009a) *Shared Leadership Underpinning of the MCLF.* Coventry: NHS Institute for Innovation and Improvement and Academy of Medical Royal Colleges.

NHS Institute for Innovation and Improvement (NHS 2009b) *Medical Leadership Competency Framework: Enhancing Engagement in Medical Leadership*, 2nd edn. London: Medical Royal Colleges.

NHS Leadership Academy (2011a) *Leadership Framework.* Coventry: NHS Institute for Innovation and Improvement.

NHS Leadership Academy (2011b) *Clinical Leadership Competency Framework.* Coventry: NHS Institute for Innovation and Improvement.

NHS Leadership Academy (2013) *Healthcare Leadership Model: The Nine Dimensions of Leadership Behaviour.* Version 1.0. Leeds: NHS Leadership Academy. Available at: www.leadershipacademy.nhs.uk/leadershipmodel (accessed 26 November 2013).

Sorensen, R., Iedema, R. and Severinsson, E. (2008) Beyond profession: nursing leadership in contemporary healthcare, *Journal of Nursing Management*, 16: 535–44.

The King's Fund (2011) *The Future of Leadership and Management in the NHS: No More Heroes.* London: The King's Fund.

Thyer, G.L. (2003) Dare to be different: transformational leadership may hold the key to reducing the nursing shortage, *Journal of Nursing Management*, 11: 73–9.

9 Conflict resolution

Caryll Overy

Introduction

This chapter will investigate how the concept of conflict resolution might apply to the contemporary paramedic professional. We begin with the origins of this supposition, but go on to relate the tangible impact of *conflict*, and its many connotations, to paramedics and their profession. In the ambulance service, conflict resolution is generally believed to be part of statutory and mandatory training (where statutory refers to a legal obligation, and mandatory refers to the employers' obligation) to protect staff from violent or aggressive behaviour while at work. There are many theories of conflict resolution, these are explained and the relevance to the paramedic profession is examined.

Historical origins of conflict resolution for ambulance personnel

The dynamic and variable nature of pre- and out-of-hospital care makes for a challenging work environment to manage. Planned outcomes of interactions with patients, relatives and the public go hand in hand with unplanned adverse interactions. Poyner and Warne (1986) suggested that for violence to occur a number of ingredients must come together (Figure 9.1).

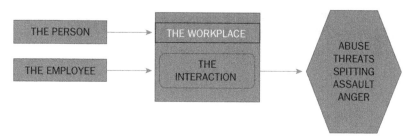

Figure 9.1 Preventing violence to staff. *Source*: Poyner and Warne (1986). © Courtesy of Solutions Training & Advisory Ltd www.solutionstraining.co.uk

Violence and aggression towards pre- and out-of-hospital practitioners is an internationally well-documented phenomenon (Boyle et al. 2007). It ranks highly as a stressor for ambulance personnel with Pozzi (1998) identifying the threat as *the worst stress factor* among pre- and out-of-hospital care providers. The Health and Safety Executive (1997) identify a number of factors that potentiate violence and aggression:

- Working alone.
- Working after normal working hours.
- Working and travelling in the community.
- Handling valuables or medication.
- Providing or withholding a service.
- Exercising authority.
- Working with people who are emotionally or mentally unstable.
- Working with people who are under the influence of drink or drugs.

Grange and Corbett (2002) detail a few more:

- Close contact without security.
- Time of day.
- Intoxication.
- Medical conditions.
- Psychiatric disorders.
- Domestic violence.

A slightly different perspective on this subject is illustrated by Bourne (2013). He considers that it is not so much why a person behaves the way they do, but what is *driving it* that is relevant. Understanding the energy behind the behaviour can play an important part when attempting to contain situations.

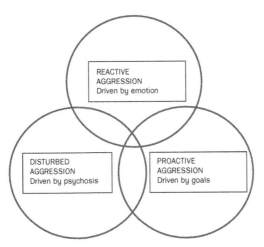

Figure 9.2   Three drivers of aggression. *Source*: Bourne (2013).

Link to the section on conflict management later in this chapter for details.

These drivers for aggressive behaviour are summed up in his *real-time* model. Each co-exists and overlaps, influencing aggressive behaviour (Figure 9.2).

Another point that is worth considering is that conflict does not have to equate to violent behaviour, it can take on a non-physical form. The National Health Service Counter Fraud and Security Management Service (NHS SMS 2004: 2) defines non-physical assault as: 'the use of inappropriate words or behaviour causing distress and/or constituting harassment'.

Violence and aggression within the workplace put employees at risk from the effects of physical and mental abuse. As employers within the United Kingdom, ambulance services have a *duty of care* to their employees. Specifically the law states, 'It shall be the duty of every employer to ensure, so far as is reasonably practicable, the health, safety and welfare at work of all his employees' (Health and Safety at Work Act 1974: section 3). There is a legal and moral obligation for employers to protect staff against both physical and non-physical assault wherever possible, consequently, the delivery of conflict resolution and personal safety instruction has become an integral part of ambulance Trusts' statutory and mandatory training provision.

In 2003, following a strategic review of security management in the Department of Health and the National Health Service, the NHS Security Management Service (NHS SMS) was created 'and charged with ensuring that all possible measures are taken to deliver a properly secure environment for all who work, or receive treatment, in the NHS' (DH 2003: 3). Recognizing the variety in content and quality of ambulance service training nationally, an NHS SMS project group has set national standards for the delivery of conflict resolution training that became live in 2007. These standards aim to 'equip frontline ambulance personnel, with the skills, knowledge and confidence to recognise, prevent and manage potentially violent situations safely and effectively' (DH 2007: 2). The result has been the provision of nationally standardized conflict resolution training, with prescribed learning outcomes for all frontline ambulance staff, that is refreshed every three years (NHS SMS 2003).

But what is conflict?

So now there is a standardized tool designed to enable ambulance staff to manage conflict safely, we need to consider what conflict actually means to us. Conflict is generally understood to be 'a struggle or clash between opposing forces or ideas' (Encarta Dictionary: English [UK]). However, this seemingly innocuous dictionary definition skims over the sociological debate of the twentieth century where defining notions have been subjective and varied. Schmidt and Kochan (1972) focus on competitive intentions and interference with each other's goals, while others define conflict as the behaviours or feelings of interdependent parties in response to potential or actual obstructions that impede one or more of the parties from achieving their goals (Deutsch 1973; Gaski 1984; Coughlan et al. 2001). Putnam and Poole (1987) divide conflict into three themes: (1) looking at inter-dependence between parties; (2) perceptions of incompatibility among parties; and (3) incompatibility of some form of interaction, whereas the *state of mind* of the parties involved is the focus for Buchanan and Huczynski (2010). This variety of considerations begins to show us the complexity of an apparently simple concept, which will be explored further.

Historically, the concept of conflict has been grouped into two broad categorizations: the *macro* and *micro* levels. Pondy (1967) championed the *macro-level*. A sociological approach focusing on formal and institutionalized causes with three main forms identified:

1. Bargaining conflict among organized interest groups.

2. Bureaucratic conflict between managers and employees.

3. Systems conflict among teams or units.

On the other hand, Nye (1973) considered the micro-level (psychological) approach or interactionist view. This concentrated on conflict within and among people, specifically intrapersonal, interpersonal, and small group behaviour. Barr and Dowding (2012) have regrouped these into three categorizations termed *levels of conflict*, see Box 9.1.

While one can broadly agree with these categorizations, it is also worth considering what the individuals are physically doing, and how they feel about doing it. This brings organizational culture and the nature of the business into play. In summary (referring to Figure 9.1), if physical or non-physical abuse is the outcome, conflict could be considered to be the situation that

---

Box 9.1 Categories or levels of conflict

INTRAPERSONAL

INTERPERSONAL

INTERGROUP

Source: Adapted from Barr and Dowding (2012).

---

is propagating it. However you choose to categorize conflict, it presents as a ubiquitous phenomenon that pervades virtually all inter-organizational activities (Lewin 1947; Dahrendorf 1959; Thomas and Kilmann 1974).

Link to Chapter 4 for more detail on organizations.

Conflict from a paramedic perspective

Read case study 9.1 to examine how conflict might look to a paramedic on a daily basis.

Case study 9.1

Fiona, the paramedic, prepares for the 12-hour early shift by getting up at 5 a.m., making lunch and then is stuck in traffic on the way to work. She arrives just on time.

Fiona is sent straight out on a category A call to an 'unconscious male', to find she is working with a long-serving colleague, Sally. No-one else on station wants to work alongside Sally. Fiona has worked with Sally previously and found her hard to work with and quite obnoxious.

On arrival to the home address, Fiona is shown by the gentleman's distressed wife to their bedroom. The patient has obviously passed away in the night and is cold, with rigor mortis present. Sally returns the equipment to the vehicle, while Fiona cares for the bereaved lady. Sally does not return to the house and does not answer her handset. After 10 minutes, Fiona decides she should check that Sally is okay, so leaves the house and returns to the vehicle. Sally is in the vehicle, listening to the radio and says she is waiting for the police to arrive. Fiona is incensed that she has left the bereaved lady to check on her colleague, who is showing gross insensitivity.

The next call is to a 'non injury fall', an elderly gentleman, who appears quite moody and questions the suitability of sending an all-female crew to him to pick him up off the floor. Fiona and Sally use their manual handling techniques and equipment and safely assist the patient to his chair. Both of them feel somewhat insulted at the gentleman's attitude to women being paramedics.

After several more calls, and getting increasingly frustrated at the lack of input from Sally, Fiona asks her what is wrong. It becomes apparent that Sally resented Fiona's university education and what she sees as a 'quick route' to paramedic status, as it has taken Sally many years.

Fiona's bad day is made worse by the lack of attention shown by the triage nurse at the local Emergency Department, when Fiona was handing over her patient. This is compounded by the negotiation required over her meal break.

Sally attends one call in the course of the shift and the patient tries to hit her. Her tone, body language and judgemental behaviour make this no surprise to Fiona. Paperwork relating to this incident needs to be completed before Fiona can finish her shift.

The shift ends and Fiona is pleased to be going home, even though she is stuck in traffic again. This gives her time for reflection on the last 13 hours. Fiona wonders if, across the course of the day, there was anything she could have done differently?

There are many events identified in case study 9.1 that are encompassed within the boundaries of conflict. Physical assault is the obvious example, but others will be identified in the following paragraphs.

Intrapersonal conflict

At the start and close of case study 9.1, Fiona, the paramedic is exposed to an area of conflict that affects her personally, as an individual. There is a need to balance commitment to work and life. With only so many hours in the day, what is done at the expense of something else? For example, our paramedic gets up early and sits in traffic when the preferred option would be to remain in bed. This example could be considered as a conflict of personal preference, or doing what you must, as opposed to what you wish. This concept can be expanded still further when looking at critical reflection, an activity recognized as a core paramedic competency (Skills for Health 2007).

Critical reflection could be considered as intrapersonal cross-examination, the asking yourself *whether you would do things differently*, raises the question of whether you actually did do the right thing. This can be a distinctly uncomfortable process and is certainly in line with our comprehension of conflict. Barr and Dowding (2012) identify this form of conflict that occurs within an individual as *intrapersonal*.

Link to Chapter 4 for more detail on organizational culture.

Interpersonal and inter-team conflict (organizational factors)

Organizational culture can play a significant role in the manifestation of conflict. Almost (2006) identifies that perceptions of injustice or disrespect can often be the cause of conflict. Fiona infers unfair treatment from management and control regarding overwork and late meal breaks. The *hard done by* perception is then reinforced by a late finish and too much paperwork, parallel sensitivities are identified within the nursing world (Van Yperen et al. 2000). Greenberg (1993) expands the concept further to include information deprivation as a conflict precursor. A perception of being *kept in the dark* can be both frustrating and insulting. Information is often only shared on a *need-to-know* basis with limited explanation as to the *why*, leaving the recipient feeling put-upon or excluded, and not valued enough to be kept informed.

However, the most significant effect of the organization is the creation of *interdependence* among team members (Putnam and Poole 1987). Interdependence relates to the reality that members of a team *need each other* in order to accomplish their work and this reliance is a stimulant for conflict. The level of conflict experienced relates proportionally to the levels of interdependence (Jehn 1992).

Link to Chapter 6 for more detail on team working and group behaviour.

Relationship conflict

The College of Paramedics (2008: 22) identifies 'commitment to team and partnership working with other professionals' as a core competency within the paramedic scope of practice. Effective practice is reliant on interpersonal communication and interdependence within teams, while embracing the equality and diversity that the participants might bring to the partnership.

Teams

Teams associated with paramedic practice might include:

- the ambulance service team, the crew and other ambulance personnel (single responders, control, other crews);

- the service user team (including patients and/or relatives and the general public);

- a multi-disciplinary team (other healthcare professionals, fire and rescue, police, coastguard, the military, etc.).

Such interdependence can propagate relationship conflict as described by Jehn (1995), where interpersonal incompatibility, personality clashes, tension, animosity and annoyance can lead to a stressful shift, as exemplified by case study 9.1. So what underpins these interdependence tensions? Fundamentally, they can be attributed to a diverse population of service users and employees. Differences in age, ethnicity, culture, gender, sexuality, and individual presentation all contribute to interpersonal interactions. Swearingen and Liberman (2004) recognized how generational diversity can lead to conflict in nursing work environments. They recognized that each generation of nurses will bring their own sets of values, beliefs, life experiences and attitudes to the workplace, not all of which will *sit well* together. This observation can also be true when applied to paramedic practice, where knowledge and systems have evolved, along with the candidates and their qualifications. While we are encouraged to embrace diversity for the added value it brings to organizations and society, it is worth considering the irony of the fact that the very element seen to enrich the workplace environment can be a driving force for disruption. Stereotypes and preconceptions inform the expectations of service users and employees, thereby if these expectations are not satisfied, relationship conflict may result. Remember the elderly gentleman from case study 9.1? He perceived that two females would be unable to manage his predicament. Additionally, Sally's outright dismissal of the value of a university education. In both these examples there is a breakdown in interpersonal relationships because of pre-conceived ideas.

Trust

The further element of *trust* must be considered if people are to work together. Mickan and Rodger (2000) and Lencioni (2002) identify trust in one another as a key component in the functionality of a team. It follows, therefore, that a lack of trust might readily contribute to a climate of conflict. Dirks and Parks (2003) suggest that trust affects our perceptions of others both through interpretation of existing actions and from previous events. By returning to case study 9.1 we observe that the crew's poor interpersonal relationship is further eroded by inadequate communication and a lack of mutual respect. Poor communication, ignoring concerns or input, or inappropriate body language and speech may well be interpreted as disrespectful (Street 2012), and they are all seen as indicators of relationship conflict (Tyler and Lind 1992; Thomas and Pondy 1977). This type of misunderstanding can be exacerbated further if there is anger, dislike or distrust present in the equation (Wall and Callister 1995).

While conflict may be underpinned by differing opinions and values which originate from cultural and social backgrounds (De Dreu and Van Lange 1995; Wall and Callister 1995), the character of a social interaction is fashioned by the dispositional traits of those involved, that is *what state of mind the individuals are in* (Friedman et al. 2000). Considering the state of mind of the individuals in case study 9.1: the *complacent* crew mate, the *irritated* crew, the *apprehensive*, anxious and violent patients and/or relatives, and the *triage* emergency department nurse. You can easily imagine that all of the individuals described are primed for conflicting interactions and unsatisfactory relationships.

Qualifications

A final consideration for the discussion on relationships are the educational qualifications of our crew. In direct response to government plans for changes to healthcare provision, expectations of paramedics' performance have risen, the delivery of paramedic education has changed. As Blaber (2008) highlighted, the Department of Health publication, *Taking Healthcare to the Patient: Transforming NHS Ambulance Services* (DH 2005), where higher education for paramedics is said to be central to achieving a modernised ambulance workforce, has had a significant effect. While integration of higher education institution (HEI) qualifications in the paramedic profession may have raised the standards of education (DH 2010) and modernized the ambulance workforce, it has also inadvertently brought about disparity and resentment.

There are currently five qualifications that are eligible for paramedic registration (HCPC 2012): with career progression and professional development firmly influenced by educational background (O'Meara 2006). The Institute of Health Care Development (IHCD) paramedic required little more than a high school education, operational experience, hard work and a glowing employment record. Now paramedic candidates must have proved themselves as academically capable by attaining high grades at 'A'-level, or equivalent, prior to commencing their paramedic studies. Consequently, the graduate paramedic already has the academic credits required for further study, whereas the IHCD paramedic must make up their academic shortfall in order to progress. The potential has thereby been raised for some registrants to feel aggrieved and undervalued, adding further fuel to the interpersonal and intrapersonal conflict fire.

As if the educational variety had not caused enough friction, Ancona (1990) identifies that variety in educational levels may also dictate how people think about and complete tasks. Individuals will approach tasks differently depending on their level of education, which in turn poses further potential for conflict and challenges for mentorship.

Link to Chapter 10 for more discussion on mentorship.

Self-reflective exercise

Make a list of predispositions toward violent behaviour and identify the drivers for each.

Task and process conflict

A further analysis of the team dynamic provides additional categorization of conflict, centred around *what needs to be done*, and how it is achieved. Jehn and Mannix (2001) recognize differences of opinion relating to the outcomes of a team task, as *task conflict*. This could be seen as challenging enough when there is a job to do, but in addition to discrepancies around the outcomes, the actual process of how to get there may also be up for debate. For example, consider how an ambulance crew might immobilize and transfer a patient: should they use a vacuum mattress or long board, or perhaps an orthopaedic stretcher? Once this decision is made, what mode of transportation would be best? Should the patient be transported by road or air? And, finally, where should the patient be transported to? Major trauma centre, or the closest emergency department? The answers to all these questions depend of course on the patient and the presenting complaint, but choices will be made based on the knowledge and experience of the healthcare professionals involved. While task conflict focuses on the content and the goals of the work, process conflict focuses on how tasks would be accomplished (Jehn 1997). Once a decision has been made, process decides *how it* can be achieved.

The paramedic scope of practice (Box 9.2) suggests that the paramedic should be equipped to manage these challenges, but what are the consequences if they are not?

Box 9.2 Scope of practice

According to the Paramedic Curriculum Guidance and Competence Framework (2008), all grades of practitioners on the paramedic pathway will be able to demonstrate:

- A knowledge and understanding of the age span of human development from preterm infant to older adult.
- Acknowledgement/understanding of individuals and groups in a broad range of settings including acute, primary and critical care settings who present with complex and challenging problems resulting from multi-pathology illness and injury.
- The integration of theory and practice and the development of creative problem solving processes.
- Effective critical reflective practice, self-evaluation and an increasing commitment to the use of evidence/research in the paramedic profession in providing optimum patient care.
- A commitment to team and partnership working with other professionals.
- A clear understanding that all registered health professionals are accountable for their clinical reasoning and resulting actions and

should be expected to give a clear rationale for the decisions enacted upon.

- An understanding of patient/client autonomy, embracing the concepts of inclusion, consent, confidentiality, equal opportunities, individual rights, diversity and empowerment of patients.
- In consultation with the patient and or their family/advocate negotiate the care pathway to the benefit of the patient.
- Arrange for appropriate and prompt referral to another health or social care professional, where the patient needs exceed the scope of practice of the paramedic.

Self-reflective exercise

Refer to the paramedic scope of practice (see Box 9.2) to help you consider how a paramedic might perceive conflict on a daily basis. Make a list of your examples.

Consequences of conflict

Almost (2006) looked at the consequences of conflict and grouped them into three areas (Figure 9.3). How might this information translate to the role of the paramedic in an ambulance Trust?

Figure 9.3 presents a broadly negative perspective, however, it is worth noting that there are both positive and negative effects to interpersonal relationships identified. However, when you consider the effects of demoralized individuals on the organization, even the apparently positive relationship points such as stronger bonds and team cohesiveness could prove damaging. A team may become more cohesive with stronger relationships, but they would be unified by the poor moral feeding their intrapersonal conflict!

Individual effects	Interpersonal relationships	Organizational effects
• Job stress • Job dissatisfaction • Absenteeism • Intent to leave • Increased grievances • Psychosomatic complaints • Negative emotions	• Negative view of others • Hostility • Avoidance • Stronger relationships • Team cohesiveness	• Reduced coordination and collaboration • Reduced productivity

Figure 9.3 Consequences of conflict. *Source:* Adapted from Almost (2006).

Link to Chapter 6 for working as a team/group dynamics and Chapter 4 for understanding the organization for more detail.

Table 9.1 highlights select question areas based on poor morale and stressors from the National Health Service (NHS) Staff Survey completed by paramedics and ambulance staff in 2012. The results suggest that ambulance personnel perceive that they are under significant stress from work-related factors. Large numbers of staff work extended hours which could potentially result in fatigue. Additionally the threat of violence, bullying and harassment from service users is real and there also appears to be a lack of confidence in senior management. It would seem that paramedics and ambulance staff experience stress, anxiety and poor morale potentiated by elements of their working environment. Consider the effects of this climate

Table 9.1 NHS Staff Survey (Ambulance Trusts)

Question	National average results
KF3. Work pressures felt by staff	3.16/5.00
KF4. Effective team working	3.31/5.00
KF5. % working extra hours	84
KF9. Support from immediate managers	3.21/5.00
KF11. % suffering work-related stress in last 12 months	44
KF13. % witnessing potentially harmful errors, near misses or incidents in last month	38
KF16. % experiencing physical violence from patients, relatives or the public in last 12 months	33
KF17. % experiencing physical violence from staff in last 12 months	3
KF18. % experiencing harassment, bullying or abuse from patients, relatives or the public in last 12 months	47
KF19. % experiencing harassment, bullying or abuse from staff in last 12 months	28
KF20. % feeling pressure in last 3 months to attend work when feeling unwell	38
KF21. % reporting good communication between senior management and staff	16
KF22. % able to contribute towards improvements at work	44
KF24. Staff recommendation of the Trust as a place to work or receive treatment	3.12/5.00
KF25. Staff motivation at work	3.56/5.00

Source: Abridged from DH (2012).

FEAR OF CONFLICT		**HEALTHY CONFLICT**

➤ Team meetings are boring
➤ Back channel politics and
   personal attacks are
   permitted
➤ Ignore controversial topics
➤ Waste time posturing and
   managing personal risk
	CONFLICT	➤ Have lively interesting
		   meetings
		➤ Extract and exploit the
		   ideals of all team members
		➤ Solve real problems quickly
		➤ Minimize politics
		➤ Put critical topics on the
		   table for discussion

Figure 9.4 Effects of conflict on a team. *Source*: Adapted from Lencioni (2002).

on the interpersonal relationships of the ambulance service, the service users and the wider NHS.

While conflict is identified as a contributor to dysfunction within a team (Lencioni 2002; Mikan and Rodger 2000), its presence is also highlighted as making a positive contribution to team effectiveness. It appears that conflict can be both intimidating and healthy, and that a team without conflict might not perform to its full potential (Figure 9.4).

Jones (1993) and De Dreu (1997) also identify the positive effects of conflict on group identity. Presence of conflict can lead to inquiry. Answers are sought, taboos are addressed and ideas are explored, contributing to an innovative dynamic climate (Nelson et al. 2011).

So at first glance, the consequences of conflict identified in Figure. 9.3 would appear to *lock* the individual, and indeed the organization into a downward spiral. However, by bringing tensions out into the open and coming to an agreement, they can actually play a positive hand in building relationships, even if the resolution is not an outright agreement but a resolve to *agree to disagree*.

Notions vary considerably when considering the concept, its effects, and the positive or negative nature of its outcomes, a lack of clarity that is hardly surprising, given the difficulty in distinguishing between episodes of conflict and the normal *give and take* of social interactions (Wrong 1979). Almost (2006) sums up this challenging enigma by depicting conflict as a multidimensional construct with both detrimental and beneficial effects.

Reflection: points to consider

How might the consequences of conflict leave the paramedic feeling about their role?

Conflict resolution

The notion of conflict resolution also seems simple enough, but as with conflict itself the concept of conflict resolution is multi-dimensional. Ramsbotham et al. (2011) identify three main presentations:

1. a practical and academic study area open for sociological and psychological debate;

2. a process that is actively used throughout the world by people with minimal consideration of the theory;

3. a peaceful outcome to a situation.

Our interests lie with the first, and as with any topic open to academic scrutiny, many angles on conflict management have been considered in the literature. Vivar (2006) suggests that those involved in the conflict should be conscious of the problem. They should take stock of the situation and apply suitable strategies to deal with it. However, this is easier said than done. Ownership is not always easy to realize. It relies on those involved having the knowledge and skills to recognize the options available. Resolution requires an informed individual or group employing an appropriate management model or strategy.

Management models

The confrontation management model is employed within current conflict resolution training (Figure 9.5). It is progressive and emphasizes that each level must be attained before moving on to the next level.

The confrontation management model (see Figure 9.5) poses escalation prevention as the starting point for conflict management. If a person is upset

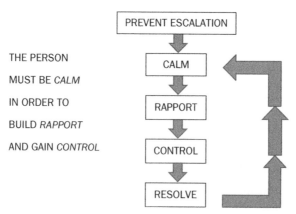

Figure 9.5 Confrontation management model. *Source:* © Courtesy of Solutions Training & Advisory Ltd www.solutionstraining.co.uk

or agitated, bombarding them with questions that do not seem relevant to them can agitate them further. It is important to remain calm, establish a rapport with the individual. If this is achieved, then you can take control of the situation and resolve issues. This cycle should de-escalate or prevent escalation of raised anxieties or agitation. It is vital that the paramedic assesses the situation quickly and accurately. This will involve picking up on cues, body language and intonation, tone and pitch of language. Awareness of problems early on, the use of this model and excellent communication skills will enable the paramedic to de-escalate the situation before it becomes troublesome.

Obtaining patient details is an essential part of the paramedic's job. However, a distressed patient or relative will not see the immediate relevance of this in resolving their crisis. This is the situation in case study 9.2, particularly when the parent has already passed on most of this information on the telephone before the ambulance arrived. Paramedics must appreciate the *bigger picture* and who the patient and family have been in contact with before their arrival, this will be indicative of how much questioning they have been subjected to previously. Remember, these are often highly charged emotional situations and the patient feels unwell, how tolerant would you be to questioning and re-questioning? If the initial contact is approached in an inappropriate fashion, the situation may become escalated making resolution more challenging. De-escalation is complex, it will require modification for each situation, and success is down to highly developed interpersonal

---

Case study 9.2 An example of escalation

It is 2 a.m. and an anxious parent telephones 111 for advice about their child who has been awake all night and is unwell.

The call handler asks the parent many questions and finally advises the parent that they will ask the ambulance service to dispatch an ambulance to their address. This advice increases the parent's anxiety, as this advice infers their child is very unwell, if they need an ambulance.

The parent puts the phone down and a car arrives outside a few minutes later, the parent was expecting an ambulance. The paramedic does a quick assessment and asks for ambulance 'back up'. The parent queries why an ambulance was not sent in the first place.

While the parent is waiting for the ambulance, the paramedic is asking more questions, many similar to all of the others.

The ambulance arrives and the child and parent are escorted to the ambulance. The crew attach the child to some equipment and ask the parent the same questions again. The parent has already answered these questions twice.

The parent loses their temper …

> ## Box 9.3   Six paradigms of human interaction
>
> - Win/Win (Both parties get what they want).
> - Win/Lose (An authoritarian approach).
> - Lose/Win (Giving in or giving up).
> - Lose/lose (Neither party is satisfied).
> - Win (You get what they want).
> - Win/Win or no deal (i.e. agree to disagree).
>
> ---
>
> *Source:* Adapted from Covey (1990).

skills. These skills enable the operator to read the signs and interpret them appropriately and are not designed to resolve the crisis but to minimize the risk of greater tension.

Bourne (2013) brings a further element to this technique in the form of *defusing skills*. He distinguishes them from de-escalation by explaining defusing skills as our professional attitude which incorporates personal and social skills and excellent customer care. Defusing skills can be used before and after de-escalation to achieve the state of calm that is required to communicate effectively and build rapport. Negotiation and influencing can then be used to gain control and achieve resolution.

The confrontation management model appears to apply a win–lose paradigm of human interaction as detailed by Covey (1990). It focuses on manipulation of the situation to gain control, and thereby impose the outcome the user desires. However, when taken within the context of the conflict management course, this model does incorporate consideration of behavioural types and explores the options of win–win outcomes (see Box 9.3).

The literature identifies five common approaches or strategies for addressing conflict resolution: competition, avoidance, accommodation, compromise and collaboration (Blake and Mouton 1968). An explanation of these strategies is offered by Thomas and Kilmann (1974) and is detailed in Table 9.2.

Thomas and Kilmann applied these strategies to a management model that looks at an individual's behaviour in conflict situations.

In addition to the five styles, they suggest two dimensions of behaviour:

1. *Assertiveness:* The extent to which an individual attempts to satisfy his or her own concerns.
2. *Cooperativeness:* The extent to which the individual attempts to satisfy the other party's concerns.

These dimensions provide the axis for the graph which is populated by the conflict handling styles. The model thus relates the conflict handling styles to preferred behaviours in conflict (Figure 9.6).

Table 9.2 Strategies to address conflict resolution

Style	Definition	Use
Competing	Pursuit of own concerns at the other person's expense, using whatever power seems appropriate to win.	Use of competition might mean standing up for your rights, defending a position you believe is correct, or trying to win.
Assertive and uncooperative. *Collaborating*	Attempting to work with the other person to find a solution that fully satisfies the concerns of both.	Use of collaboration might involve digging into an issue to identify the underlying concerns of the two individuals to find an alternative that meets the needs of both.
Assertive and cooperative, both sets of concerns. *Compromising*	The object is to find an expedient, mutually acceptable solution that partially satisfies both parties.	Compromise might mean splitting the difference, exchanging concessions, or seeking a quick middle-ground position. Intermediate in both assertiveness and cooperativeness.
Avoiding	One does not immediately pursue own concerns or those of the other person or address the conflict.	Avoidance might take the form of diplomatically sidestepping an issue, postponing an issue until a better time, or simply withdrawing from a threatening situation.
Unassertive and uncooperative. *Accommodating*	Neglecting own concerns to satisfy concerns of the other person.	Use of accommodation might take the form of selfless generosity or charity, obeying another person's order when asked. Unassertive and cooperative you would prefer not to, or yielding to another's point of view.

Source: Thomas and Kilmann (1974).

So which of the five suggested strategies should be used? The negative reputation of conflict can be compounded by the methods employed to manage it. Conflict management training for paramedics focuses on the negative outcomes of conflict and how to de-escalate or escape. Conflict is depicted as dangerous and employees must be equipped to manage the risk. The syllabus

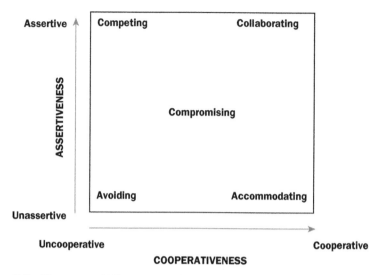

Figure 9.6 Thomas and Kilmann's model of conflict handling (1974).

has overriding themes that strengthen this negativity, including the notion that conflict is dangerous, and employees must be protected against it. However, this impression is not so much the fault of the training programme itself, it is more the fault of how it is employed. There is a pre-conception of the learning outcomes prior to attendance. Many believe that this statutory and mandatory training will deliver physical self-defence skills. They also take the practical elements as an opportunity to exhibit physical strength and competitiveness: who will be able to grip the tightest or topple the heaviest person? This is not directly the fault of the individuals involved, but is down to both human nature and organizational culture of taking control, strength is power, survival of the fittest, brute strength and ignorance and many more clichés. The discerning professional might adopt a more pragmatic attitude considering negotiation, reasoning and collaboration as learning outcomes.

Link to Chapter 4 Understanding the organization.

These are two extreme stereotypical examples, but what is the difference between them and how did it come about? Fundamentally it is about what they know and understand about themselves, others and interactions between, see Box 9.4. Who you are prescribes not only what you perceive conflict management to be, but also how you will go about managing conflict.

There are a multitude of factors that might influence the approach you adopt, including: gender (Valentine 2004), age and experience (Swearingen and Liberman 2004), social and cultural influences (De Dreu and Van Lange 1995; Wall and Callister 1995), education and position within an organization

---

Box 9.4   Conflict handling tool kit

For making decisions on conflict handling style to be made there must be:

- knowledge of one's self ;
- knowledge of the personal style preference;
- an ability to read a situation;
- knowledge of styles available;
- knowledge of the best fit;
- ability to communicate utilising the appropriate style.

(Hendel et al. 2005), state of mind (Friedman et al. 2000), and personality (Whitworth 2008), along with combinations of these factors (Sportsman and Hamilton 2007).

This situation is further complicated by a suggestion that we should alter our conflict handling skills depending on who we are dealing with (Whetten et al. 2000). Certain conflict handling styles might not be amicably paired with particular types of conflict, so we must be able to read the situation and modify our response accordingly.

Whetton et al. (2000) suggest that there are four main considerations when applying a style for successful resolution:

1. The importance of the outcome, does it matter or not? (Considering the conflict a paramedic might meet, it could literally be a life or death situation.)

2. The importance of the relationship. (Again, with paramedic practice, the relationship is of high importance. There is little hope for compliance in this matter or any future interactions if the relationship has broken down.)

3. What is the position you are coming from? (Are you a supervisor or manager or a peer?)

4. And finally how much time do you have? (Again, for the paramedic, the incident could be time-critical where every second counts.)

The capacity to resolve conflict is determined by the skills and resources available (Tidwell 1998), so are all ambulance employees equipped with this tool kit? The answer is, probably not.

Conflict: a leadership perspective

Closer inspection of conflict resolution skills identifies many similarities with the Skills For Health (SFH) Health Functional map (2007), from which the National Occupational Standards (NOS) have been drawn. These standards lay down the competences that the paramedic scope of practice (Box 9.2) refers to. Registered paramedics should therefore have the skills required, however, for this to be the case the paramedic curriculum that furnished their registration would need to have been developed in conjunction with the NOS.

This is certainly the case with HCPC (Approved) and College of Paramedics (Endorsed) courses, so those educated through HEI programmes should have the fundamental skills required, but the paramedics pre-dating this time may not. Whether previous exposure exists or not, further advance is always valuable for continuing professional development.

The skills identified can also be mapped to domains 1 and 2 of NHS Leadership Academy Clinical Leadership Competency Framework (Leadership Academy, 2011) (see Boxes 9.5 and 9.6). The NHS Leadership Academy has been established to define national standards for leadership within the NHS.

Box 9.5   NHS Leadership Academy domain 1

1.0 Demonstrating personal qualities

1.1 Leaders **develop self awareness**: being aware of their own values, principles and assumptions and by being able to learn from experiences.

Competent leaders:

- Recognise and articulate their own values and principles, understanding how these may differ from those of other individuals and groups
- Identify their own strengths and limitations, the impact of their behaviour on others, and the effect of stress on their own behaviour
- Identify their own emotions and prejudices and understand how these can affect their judgement and behaviour
- Obtain, analyse and act on feedback from a variety of sources

1.2 Leaders **manage themselves**: organising and managing themselves while taking account of the needs and priorities of others.

Competent leaders:

- Manage the impact of their emotions on their behaviour with consideration of the impact on others
- Are reliable in meeting their responsibilities and commitments to consistently high standards
- Ensure that their plans and actions are flexible, and take account of the needs and work patterns of others
- Plan their workload and activities to fulfil work requirements and commitments, without compromising their own health

1.3 Leaders actively engage in **continuing personal development**: learning through participating in continuing professional development and from experience and feedback.

Competent leaders:

- Actively seek opportunities and challenges for personal learning and development
- Acknowledge mistakes and treat them as learning opportunities
- Participate in continuing professional development activities
- Change their behaviour in the light of feedback and reflection

1.4 Leaders **act with integrity**: behaving in an open, honest and ethical manner.

Competent leaders:

- Uphold personal and professional ethics and values, taking into account the values of the organisation and respecting the culture, beliefs and abilities of individuals
- Communicate effectively with individuals, appreciating their social, cultural, religious and ethnic backgrounds and their age, gender and abilities
- Value, respect and promote equality and diversity
- Take appropriate action if ethics and values are compromised

Source: Leadership Academy (2012).

It encourages a diversity of leadership styles and focuses on the importance of patient and staff engagement in leading quality improvement (The King's Fund 2012). The Leadership Framework is based on the concept that leadership is not restricted to people who hold designated management and traditional leader roles, but in fact is most successful wherever there is a shared responsibility for the success of the organization, services or care being delivered.

This puts leadership responsibilities firmly in the hands of paramedics and opens the doors of opportunity for development in this area. It seems that inadvertently by developing conflict handling skills, we will also develop leadership skills, and development of leadership skills will assist with conflict management.

Self-reflective exercise:
- Consider your own conflict and leadership skills. How might you develop these skills through personal and professional CPD? Take these considerations to form the basis of your next *personal development review.*

Box 9.6   NHS Leadership academy domain 2

2.0 Working with others

2.1 Leaders **develop networks**: working in partnership with patients, carers, service users and their representatives, and colleagues within and across systems to deliver and improve services.

Competent leaders:

- Identify opportunities where working in collaboration with others within and across networks can bring added benefits
- Create opportunities to bring individuals and groups together to achieve goals
- Promote the sharing of information and resources
- Actively seek the views of others

2.2 Leaders **build and maintain relationships**: listening, supporting others, gaining trust and showing understanding.

Competent leaders:

- Listen to others and recognise different perspectives
- Empathise and take into account the needs and feelings of others
- Communicate effectively with individuals and groups, and act as a positive role model
- Gain and maintain the trust and support of colleagues

Source: Leadership Academy (2012).

The Healthcare Leadership Model (2013) does little to expand upon the 2011 Leadership Framework, in respect of conflict resolution. While it is recognized that version 1.0 of the new model will be continually evaluated and updated, as it remains current, it reflects the climate of the NHS and the constant changes of the service, the dimension 'Engaging the team' is very brief. When working with teams, conflict (both positive and negative) will occur, this is not acknowledged or referred to in the 2013 Healthcare Leadership Model.

Conclusion

Should we view conflict resolution as a practical health and safety tool or as a developmental opportunity for leadership skills? The traditional ambulance view is *to fix* the problem with some training. Conflict resolution training has been adopted to address the Health and Safety Obligations of the employer, and while it introduces the knowledge and skills required, it is too time-constrained to effectively develop the candidates to the full potential.

Management development packages that are developed through government incentives have started to address the internal skills deficit. The Professional, Statutory and Regulatory bodies (PSRBs) dictate what should be included within HEI paramedic science programmes. Sociology, ethics, interpersonal skills communication are all explored to a far greater extent than was ever an option with traditional paramedic education, and in so doing Higher Education is facilitating the development of professional leaders in pre- and out-of-hospital healthcare.

Both the organization and its employees must apply positive measures relating to continuing personal and professional development to move on. While the employer has a responsibility to ensure the health and safety of their staff, it is the employee's responsibility to practise their professional commitment to lifelong learning.

Chapter key points

- The nature of ambulance service work will expose staff to varieties of conflict.
- Organizations and employees will encounter various types of conflict during the course of their duties.
- Before conflict can be fully understood or resolved it is important that the theory of aggression is understood.
- There are various categories of conflict, such as intrapersonal, interpersonal, inter-team and relationship.
- In addition to relationship conflict, the role and organisation can be the cause of conflict for the individual.
- Conflict has consequences for the individual, team, the efficiency and effectiveness of the organization.
- There are many conflict resolution management models and some key factors that are useful.
- Leaders will encounter conflict and will have to help resolve conflict to the satisfaction of all parties.
- A knowledge of the models available should help leaders develop their skills in conflict resolution as part of their continuing professional development.

References and suggested reading

Almost, J. (2006) Conflict within nursing work environments: concept analysis, *Journal of Advanced Nursing*, 53(4): 444–53.

Ancona, D. (1990) Outward bound: strategies for team survival in the organisation, *Academy of Management Journal*, 33: 334–65.

Barr, J. and Dowding, L. (2012) *Leadership in Health Care*, 2nd edn. London. Sage.

Blaber, A.Y. (ed.) (2012) *Foundations for Paramedic Practice: A Theoretical Perspective*, 2nd edn. Maidenhead: Open University Press.

Blake, R. R. and Mouton J. S. (1964) *The Managerial Grid*. Houston, TX: Gulf.

Bourne, I. (2013) *Facing Danger in the Helping Professions: A Skilled Approach*. Maidenhead: Open University Press.

Boyle, M., Koritsas, S., Coles, J. and Stanley, J. (2007) A pilot study of workplace violence towards paramedics. *Emergency Medical Journal*, 24: 760–3.

Buchanan, D. and Huczynski, A. (2010) *Organizational Behavior*. London: Financial Times/Prentice Hall.

CoP College of Paramedics (2008) *Paramedic Curriculum Guidance and Competence framework* 2nd edn. Derby: College of Paramedics.

Coughlan, A., Anderson, E., Stern, L. and El-Ansary, A.I. (2001) *Marketing Channels*, 6th edn. Englewood Cliffs, NJ: Prentice Hall.

Covey, S. (1990) *The 7 Habits of Highly Effective People: Powerful lessons in Personal Change*. New York: Fireside.

Dahrendorf, R. (1959) *Class and Class Conflict in Industrial Society*. Stanford, CA: Stanford University Press.

Department of Health (2003) *Protecting Your NHS: A Professional Approach to Managing Security in the NHS*. Available at: http://www.nhsbsa.nhs.uk/Documents/sms_strategy.pdf (accessed 17 July 2013).

Department of Health (2005) *Taking Healthcare to the Patient: Transforming NHS Ambulance Services*. London: DH Publications.

Department of Health (2007) *Protecting Your NHS: Implementing Learning Outcomes in Conflict Resolution for NHS Ambulance Services: Frequently Asked Questions*. Available at: http://www.nhsbsa.nhs.uk/SecurityManagement/Documents/ambulance_crt_faq.pdf (accessed 17 July 2013).

Department of Health (2010) *Liberating the NHS: Developing the Healthcare Workforce*. London: DH Publications.

De Dreu, C.K.W. (1997) Productive conflict: the importance of conflict management and conflict issues, in C.K.W. De Dreu and E. Van de Vliert (eds) *Using Conflict in Organisations*. London: Sage, pp. 9–22.

De Dreu, C.K.W. and Van Lange, P. A. (1995) The impact of social value orientations on negotiator cognition and behavior. *Personality and Social Psychology*, 25: 2049–66.

Deutsch, M. (1973) *The Resolution of Conflict*. New Haven, CT: Yale University Press.

Dirks, K.T. and McLean Parks, J. (2003) Conflicting stories: The state of the science of conflict, in J. Greenberg (ed.) *Organizational Behavior: The State of the Science*, 2nd edn. Hillsdale NJ: Lawrence Earlbaum Associates, pp. 283–324.

Encarta® World English Dictionary [UK. Edition] © & (P) 1998–2007 Microsoft Corporation. All rights reserved. Developed for Microsoft by Bloomsbury Publishing Plc.

Fisher, R.J. (2000) Intergroup conflict, in M. Deutsch and P. T. Coleman (eds) *The Handbook of Conflict Resolution*. San-Francisco, CA: Jossey-Bass Publishers.

Friedman, R.A., Tidd, S.T., Currall, S.C. and Tsai, J. C. (2000) What goes around comes around: the impact of personal conflict style on work conflict and stress. *International Journal of Conflict Management*, 11: 32–55.

Gaski, J.F. (1984) The theory of power and conflict in channels of distribution, *Journal of Marketing*, 48: 9–29.

Golnaz, S. (2012) Conflict's here. What now? *Industrial Management*, 54(3): 20–5.

Grange, J.T. and Corbett, S.W. (2002) Violence against emergency services personnel, *Pre-hospital Emergency Care*, 6(2):186–90.

Greenberg, J. (1993) The social side of fairness: interpersonal and informational classes of organisational justice, in R. Cropanzano (ed.) *Justice in the Workplace:*

Approaching Fairness in Human Resource Management. Hillsdale, NJ: Lawrence Erlbaum Associates, pp. 79–103.

Health and Safety Executive (1997) Violence and aggression to staff in health services. Available at: http://www.hse.gov.uk/pubns/priced/violenceinhealth.pdf (accessed 17 July 2013).

Health Care Professions Council (2012) Register of approved programmes. Available at: http://www.hpcuk.org/education/programmes/register/index.asp?Education ProviderID=all&StudyLevel=all&ModeOfStudyID=all&professionID=10&Submit. x=38&Submit.y=15 (accessed 17 July 2013).

Hendel, T., Fish, M. and Galon, V. (2005) Leadership style and choice of strategy in conflict management among Israeli nurse managers in general hospitals, *Journal of Nursing Management*, 13: 137–46.

Jehn, K.A. (1992) The impact of intra-group conflict on group effectiveness: a multi-method examination of the benefits and detriments of conflict. Unpublished doctoral dissertation, Northwestern University Evanston, IL.

Jehn, K.A. (1995) A multi-method examination of the benefits and detriments of intra-group conflict, *Administrative Science Quarterly*, 40: 256–82.

Jehn, K.A. (1997) A qualitative analysis of conflict types and dimensions in organizational groups. *Administrative Science Quarterly*, 42: 530–57.

Jehn, K.A. and Mannix, E. (2001) The dynamic nature of conflict: a longitudinal study of intragroup conflict and performance, *Academy of Management Journal*, 44: 238–51.

Jones, K. (1993) Confrontation: methods and skills, *Nursing Management*, 24(5): 68–70.

Lencioni, P. (2002) *The Five Dysfunctions of a Team: A Leadership Fable.* San Francisco: Jossey-Bass.

Lewin, K. (1947) Frontiers in group dynamics, *Human Relations*, 1(1): 1–45.

Maple, G. (1987) Early intervention: some issues in co-operative team work, *Australian Occupational Therapy Journal*, 34(4): 145–51.

Mickan, S. and Rodger, S. (2000) Characteristics of effective teams: a literature review, *Australian Health Review*, 23(3): 201–8.

Nelson, D.L., Armstrong, A., Condie, J. and Quick, J. C. (2011) *ORGB*. Cengage Learning.

NHS Leadership Academy (2013) *Healthcare Leadership Model: The Nine Dimensions of Leadership Behaviour.* Version 1.0. Leeds: NHS Leadership Academy. Available at: www.leadershipacademy.nhs.uk/leadershipmodel (accessed 26 November 2013).

NHS SMS (2003) *Conflict Resolution Refresher Training: Implementing Refresher Training.* London: NHS.

NHS Security Management Service (2004). Non physical assault explanatory notes. London: NHSSMS. Available at: http://www.nhsbsa.nhs.uk/SecurityManagement/Documents/non_physical_assault_notes.pdf (accessed 17 July 2013).

NHS Staff Survey (2012) Ambulance Trusts. Available at: http://nhsstaffsurveys.com/cms/index.php?page=ambulance-trusts-2 (accessed 17 July 2013).

Nye, R.D. (1973) *Conflict among Humans.* New York: Springer.

O'Meara, P. (2006) Searching for paramedic academics: vital for our future, but nowhere to be seen!, *Journal of Emergency Primary Health Care*, 4(4): Article 1. Available at: http://ro.ecu.edu.au/jephc/vol4/iss4/1 (accessed 17 July 2013).

Pondy, L.R. (1967) Organisational conflict: concepts and models, *Administrative Science Quarterly*, 12: 296–320.

Poyner, B. and Warne, C. (1986) Preventing violence to staff, cited in *Conflict Resolution for Ambulance Staff: Trainee's Workbook.* (2010). Solutions Training and Advisory Limited, p. 3.

Pozzi, C. (1998) Exposure of pre-hospital providers to violence and abuse, *Journal of Emergency Nursing*, 24: 320–3.

Putnam, L. and Poole, M. (1987) Conflict and negotiation, in F. Jablin, L. Putnam, K. Roberts and L. Porter (eds) *Handbook of Organizational Communication: An Interdisciplinary Perspective*. Thousand Oaks, CA: Sage, pp. 459–99.

Rahim, M.A. and Magner, N. (1995) Confirmatory factor analysis of the styles of handling interpersonal conflict: first-order factor model and its invariance across groups, *Journal of Applied Psychology*, 80: 122–32.

Ramsbotham, O., Miall, H. and Woodhouse, T. (2011) *Contemporary Conflict Resolution*. Cambridge: Polity Press.

Schmidt, S.M. and Kochan, T.A. (1972) Conflict: toward conceptual clarity, *Administrative Science Quarterly*, 17(3): 359–70.

Skills for Health. (2007) *Health Functional Map*. Available at: http://www.skillsforhealth.org.uk/page/competence-application-tools (accessed 17 July 2013).

Sportsman, S. and Hamilton, P. (2007) Conflict management styles in the health professions, *Journal of Professional Nursing*, 23(3): 157–66.

Street, P.A. (2012) Interpersonal communication: a foundation of practice, in A.Y. Blaber (ed). *Foundations for Paramedic Practice: A Theoretical Perspective*, 2nd edn. Maidenhead: McGraw-Hill/Open University Press.

Swearingen, S. and Liberman, A. (2004) Nursing generations: an expanded look at the emergence of conflict and its resolution, *The Health Care Manager*, 23(1): 54–64.

The King's Fund (2012) *Leadership and Engagement for Improvement in the NHS: Together We Can*. London. The King's Fund.

Thomas, K.W. and Kilmann, W. (1974) Conflict and conflict management, in M.D. Dunnette (ed.) *Handbook of Industrial and Organizational Psychology*. Chicago: Rand McNally, pp. 889–935.

Thomas, K.W. and Pondy, L.R. (1977) Toward an 'intent' model of conflict management among principal parties, *Human Relations Journal*, 12: 1089–102.

Tidwell, A.C. (1998) The challenge of conflict resolution, in A.C. Tidwell (ed.) *Conflict Resolved? A Critical Assessment of Conflict Resolution*. London: Continuum, pp. 1–10.

Tyler, T.R. and Lind, E.A. (1992) A relational model of authority in groups, in M. Zanna (ed.) *Advances in Experimental Social Psychology*. New York: Academic Press, pp. 115–92.

Valentine, P.E. (2001) A gender perspective on conflict management strategies of nurses, *Journal of Nursing Scholarship*, 33(1): 69–74.

Van Yperen, N., Hagedoorn, M., Zweers, M. and Postma, S. (2000) Injustice and employees' destructive responses: the mediating role of state negative affect, *Social Justice Research*, 13(3): 291–312.

Vivar, C.G. (2006) Putting conflict management into practice: a nursing case study, *Journal of Nursing Management*, 14: 201–6.

Wall, J. and Callister, R. (1995) Conflict and its management, *Journal of Management*, 21: 515–58.

Whetten, D.A., Cameron, K.S. and Woods, M. (2000) *Developing Management Skills for Europe*. Reading, MA: Addison-Wesley.

Whitworth, B.S. (2008) Is there a relationship between personality type and preferred conflict-handling styles? An exploratory study of registered nurses in southern Mississippi, *Journal of Nursing Management*, 16: 921–32.

Wrong, D. (1979) *Power: Its Forms, Bases and Uses*. Oxford: Basil Blackwell.

Mentorship and preceptorship

Kevin Barrett and Linda Nelson

Introduction

Preceptorship and mentorship are two mechanisms that support learning in the practice setting and though it is acknowledged that there are certain overlaps between the two, e.g. the attributes of appropriate personnel who support learning (Gopee 2011: 9), there are key differences that exist between preceptorship and mentorship and it is important that these differences are highlighted so that Mentors and Preceptors are clear about their role.

Mentorship

Terminology

The role of supporting and supervising clinical students in practice is central to healthcare both in the UK and abroad. The term used to identify this role in practice varies between *practice placement educator* – which the Health and Care Professions Council (HCPC) use for the 16 professions it regulates – and *mentorship*, which is employed by most other healthcare professions, notably midwifery and nursing. The term *mentorship* will be used here, given its cross-disciplinary usage, and because it appears to be the term of choice in much of the recent paramedic literature.

Together with preceptorship, the practice of mentoring is found across the full scope of paramedic practice for students in pre-registration programmes and has long seen calls for deliberate provision for newly qualified paramedics, too (Pointer 2001). It is also needed as practitioners begin to undertake specialist clinical, educational, managerial and research roles and further engage with their on-going continuing personal and professional development (CPPD). Some variance in understanding of what the role, overall, entails is noted, despite the longstanding history of mentorship (Sibson and Mursell 2010a). It is noteworthy that the HCPC does not provide an especially clear delineation of what the responsibilities are, nor what formal preparation a mentor ought to have. The HCPC Standards of Education and Training standard 5 states that:

> 5.7 Practice placement educators must have relevant knowledge, skills and experience.
>
> 5.8 Practice placement educators must undertake appropriate practice placement educator training.
>
> 5.9 Practice placement educators must be appropriately registered, unless other arrangements are agreed.
>
> (HCPC 2012a: 8)

Nonetheless, the above document does see mentorship as indispensable to clinical practice placements and the HCPC (2012 b) has identified mentoring specifically as a form of continuing personal and professional development (CPPD). Certainly, it meets their stipulation that CPD activities:

- are a mixture of learning activities relevant to current or future practice

- contribute to the quality of practice and service delivery (HCPC 2012b: 2).

In paramedic practice specifically, the role – now seen as an essential one to help manage changes both in the demands of practice itself and the shifting demographics of student paramedics – is undergoing calls for a uniformed, structured *mentorship accreditation* to be introduced nationally (Jones et al. 2012). Historically, then, we are currently at a good point to consider an overview of mentorship.

Mentorship: an overview

To date, a huge amount has been written about mentorship and most elements of this multi-faceted phenomenon have been reviewed (Gopee 2011). Although it is beyond the reach of a single chapter to cover all of these appropriately, those aspects that are emergent within contemporary paramedic practice and that impact most noticeably upon the maturation of paramedic practice as a profession will be the focus here, alongside some suggestions for the development of practice assessment, namely:

- the *new* type of paramedic student requiring mentor support;

- promoting and addressing professional attitudes;

- supporting struggling students;

- working relationships with Higher Education Institutions.

It is now well recognized that the paramedic profession is moving steadily towards an educational model as opposed to the vocational training model of preparing new registrants (College of Paramedics 2008). This is in part due to the increased demands and increasing complexity of the paramedic's workload (Armitage 2011) and an education provided in Higher Education Institutions (HEI) is viewed as a necessary one to equip paramedics with the complex decision-making and underpinning knowledge base required to respond to clinical practice as it continues to evolve (Ryan and Halliwell 2012). This move to educational programmes in HEIs is happening extremely quickly: at the time of writing, of the 72 HCPC approved paramedic programmes in the UK, 62 are already being delivered in HEIs with 15 Institute of Health Care Development (IHCD) programmes still operational and two courses being provided by private companies (HCPC 2013).

It is the view of the professional body – the College of Paramedics – that the entry threshold to the HCPC register should be BSc (Hons) degree level (College of Paramedics 2013a). Whilst this present move into HEI led education will bring the profession into line with the other 15 professions regulated by the IICPC, it will introduce both a *sea change* in the student body as well as a significant transformation of the traditional culture of paramedic practice. It is important for this to be recognized and addressed by mentors.

Link to Chapter 6 for more discussion about team dynamics.

The changing demographics of students

Traditionally, a student paramedic would have already been in a clinical role within the ambulance service prior to commencing an *in-house* or apprenticeship-style training programme, typically accredited by the IHCD. The student would probably have been a technician and possibly also had some experience of patient transport services. This infers that the student would have some insight into how the ambulance service operates, as well as have a realistic sense of what the paramedic role itself entails and the type of work that is normally met. It also suggests that the youngest student paramedics would be in their early twenties.

Courses offered at HEIs are accessed via application to the Universities and Colleges Admissions Service (UCAS) and applicants may be as young as 18. While many HEIs will require some clinical experience from a candidate before they are interviewed, it is often not required that this be within an ambulance service or pre-hospital setting. Indeed, not all ambulance services offer the opportunity to observe paramedics at work. This can mean that the students are young, potentially 18–19 years old – compared to the *traditional* student paramedic – and possibly lack genuine insight into the realities and demands of the job. There is an immediate impact upon the mentoring role of the registered paramedic in this light. One recent development within HEIs is the revision of interview practices to better identify candidates who might be well suited to the scope of experience that will come with the role and the personal and professional attributes needed (Le May et al. 2007; Eva et al. 2004).

The stresses of accident and emergency work and coping differences

It needs to be acknowledged by mentors that front-line accident and emergency work *does* present high mental and physical occupational stresses (Bower et al. 2012). In fact, as averaged over the last three years (2009/10–2011/12), of all the industries in Great Britain, healthcare work has the highest estimated prevalence rate of work-related psychological stress (Health and Safety Executive 2013) as well as the highest estimated prevalence rates of back-related musculoskeletal disorders (HSE 2012). Furthermore, within the healthcare industry itself, ambulance personnel were the staff group with the highest average sickness absence rate and, among the many different types of organizations represented, Ambulance Trusts had the highest average sickness absence rates (HSE 2013). These findings are reflected internationally, too, for paramedics (Hegg-Deloye et al. 2014).

It is also the case that paramedics cope with many of these stresses in predominantly informal ways (Mildenhall 2012a) which often rely on off stage support such as spouses or partners (Williams 2013), both of which mean that the managing of these stresses does not always happen overtly or directly within a clinical shift. The role modelling that this can present to younger or at least less clinically experienced students can mean that they are unsure how to express or process these same experiences during a shift. It may also be the case that many students lack a spouse/partner with whom to debrief when away from clinical placement (Williams 2013) and university students may be living away from their established personal support networks. Alongside the changes in the age of student paramedics is the increasing number of women – the culture of the ambulance service has been, at least until recently, predominantly male (Williams 2012). These are both examples of shifts in the *social demographic* that paramedic mentors will meet in their role and point to an element of mentoring that lies beyond teaching and assessing the required psycho-motor skill sets and more to exemplifying sane and mature responses to what is a demanding and some-times misunderstood allied health profession role. Calls for increased for-malization of *occupational support* to respond to potential clinical stresses are emerging within paramedic practice (Mildenhall 2012b).

> **Link to Chapter 4 for more detail on the role organizations have in providing support for employees**

Social and cultural issues of mentorship

These social and cultural issues are highly relevant: almost all of the courses providing paramedic education in the UK stipulate that the course is weighted 50 per cent towards practice and initial studies of student para-medics' early experiences tell us that they place a stronger reliance on the support and identity that they find in practice placements than they do on their identity as university students (Jones et al. 2010). There is a process of *acculturation* noted within contemporary paramedic research that mentors are absolutely at the heart of, as they have a primary impact on students' development within the culture of practice (Donaghy 2011). These cultural influences are in addition to the direct impact that mentors are known to have on clinical practices (Armstrong 2010).

This aspect of the role of mentor – that of role model or even *guide* through current culture and praxis – has already been noted in terms of the devel-opment of the professional behaviours that will influence paramedic pro-fessionalism altogether (Woollard 2009). Considered an *ethical* aspect of mentorship practice, role-modelling has been detailed as a fundamental and critical function – beyond the supervision of knowledge-base acquisition or skills competence (King et al. 2009). So, although students may have clear guidance on the behaviours and professional standards expected of them (HCPC 2012c), it is we as mentors who need to be able to communicate and embody these professional attitudes, alongside addressing the required skills and knowledge. Students place considerable value on good role mod-els, articulating that this is a singular influence on their own development and confidence as clinicians (Donaldson and Carter 2005).

Attitude is an area that is potentially harder to measure in a student compared to a skills performance or knowledge level which can often be calculated with a percentage mark. Nonetheless, it comprises an essential component of the well-established taxonomy that is typically used to encompass the expectations of professional competencies: knowledge, skills and attitudes. The HCPC state that, in tandem with the proficiencies detailed for registrants in the 'Standards of Proficiency: Paramedics', 'We also expect you to keep to our *standards of conduct, performance and ethics*, which are published in a separate document' (HCPC 2012d: 5).

It is significant that some 92 per cent of complaints received by the HCPC over the recent eight-year period involved conduct-related incidents (van der Gaag and Donaghy 2013). The support and development of professional attitudes, then, are of paramount importance to the profession and much will lie in the exemplifying of these behaviours within the mentorship role.

One potential future development could, conceivably, be that paramedic mentorship undertakes a similar path to that of midwifery in that pre-registration students be assessed in practice by *sign-off* mentors prior to registration with the regulatory body (NMC 2006). This is to say that the mentor is verifying that, in their professional judgement, the student has met the required proficiencies to register as a paramedic. Some of these proficiencies, of course, relate to professional attitude. This has a significant additional gravity to it as the sign-off mentor is accountable in their sign-off decision to the HCPC. Of note here is the fact that the student/new registrant is the one responsible for and accountable for their own behaviours and decisions, etc.: the sign-off mentor is *not* being held to account for the new registrant's mistakes in practice, if there were any. It is an interesting healthcare profession's development in terms of the rigour demonstrated in confirming eligibility for registration. However, given that much of the role will remain involved with managing *professionalism* – and that significant numbers of mentors report that they lack confidence in managing poor behaviour, for example (Brown et al. 2012) – it is necessary to consider some related issues here.

Challenges for mentors

Despite the vagaries of the term *competence* (Cassidy 2009), a key function of mentors is to assess students' performance and capabilities in practice (Sibson and Mursell 2010b) and it is to them that the difficulties of addressing poor performance, supporting those students who are in danger of failing elements of their course and making summative decisions about progress on the course overall will fall. In her seminal work on the challenges faced by mentors in failing students in practice, Duffy (2003) underscored the difficulties of failing students due to their *attitude*. This appears still to be the case (Gainsbury 2010).

Almost inevitably, mentors will meet a student who is struggling in some aspect of their work and it has been recognized that there is a wide range of areas that constitute the early signs of a student who is at risk of failing or developing poor professional attitudes; these will include personal and professional concerns as well as skills and knowledge deficits (Duffy 2003; Skingley et al. 2007). Many of these manifestations can be vague and not easy to pin down, document or provide feedback about, some are listed in Table 10.1:

Table 10.1 Potential indicators of poor professional attitude

Indicator	Examples	Possible responses
Communication	Inappropriate language, interrupting patients or relatives, condescension Potentially intimidating or disinterested body language	Enquire about the underlying reasons – document concerns if appropriate. Advise the student about how they may be coming across to others. This is a potentially sensitive area as many people can feel that feedback about communication is a personal issue as opposed to professional.
Timekeeping	Lateness or absences and poor communication with mentor or station about reasons why	Enquire about the underlying reasons – document concerns if appropriate. Document on student's time sheet each instance of lateness Liaise with HEI – typically the personal tutor – each instance of absence Agree an action plan with a time line for review of attendance patterns
Appearance	'Borderline' or needing prompts to wear hair or uniform in a professional manner	Enquire about the underlying reasons – document concerns if appropriate. Agree an action plan with a time line for review. Liaise with HEI – typically the personal tutor if no improvement – representing the NHS or the HEI unprofessionally could be grounds to temporarily suspend practice.
Lack of focus at work	Self-absorption. Continual discussion about personal/ social concerns	Enquire about the underlying reasons – document if appropriate. Suggest student liaise with personal tutor or student services at HEI. Possible liaison with Occupational Health or HEI
Lack of interest at work	Not taking initiative or taking advantage of learning situations	Enquire about the underlying reasons – document if appropriate.
Poor insight into areas of under-development (knowledge, skills, attitude)	Unaware when asked that there is a perceived concern about levels of knowledge or skills or professionalism	Provide concrete examples of concerns Liaise with personal tutor: possible tripartite meeting to consider an action plan
Poor response to feedback	No appreciable change in behaviour or approach to clinical practice	Enquire about the underlying reasons – document if appropriate. Liaise with personal tutor: possible tripartite meeting to consider an action plan.

Reflection: points to consider

- What other criteria might alert you to someone that is not meeting the professional expectations of a student paramedic?
- What might you expect of a student in terms of attitude in year 1? In year 2? In year 3?

One other instance of professional behaviour may be the use of social media sites by students (Davies 2013). Student paramedics will often have many *interesting* stories that they want to share and fail to appreciate the constraints that employers or the HCPC place on this form of communication (HCPC 2013b).

A demonstration of good practice that is consistently forwarded in the literature is that concerns are attended to and documented as early as possible, as students are often alerted late in their course about inadequacies (Duffy 2003) and this is unfair on the student. A discussion with colleagues can be supportive, as can liaison with the student's personal tutors at the university, as colleagues may have insight or information unavailable to oneself at any given point. One formal mechanism that aims to facilitate discussion is the *tripartite meeting*: student, mentor and HEI representative meet to consider each other's perspective on an issue. It is wise to brief the student on the purpose of the meeting beforehand as it is possible for students to feel *outnumbered* by the other staff present, but action plans arising from these meetings do address a rounded view of a situation.

The actual discussion that is needed with students that are presenting some form of attitude-related concern is often quite complicated and can address sensitive issues that are unexpected. Table 10.2 is a consideration of some facets that support an approach to these difficult conversations.

Reflection: points to consider

- What disadvantages might there be surrounding 'privacy'?
- What solutions might there be here?
- What might the support be referred to in 'Planning ahead' entail? For the student? For you?

Support mechanisms for mentor and student

It should be highlighted here that it is impossible to predict what degree of support any individual student may need. Recent studies into students'

Table 10.2 Preparing for a difficult interview

Preparation	Comments
1. **P**rior Agreement	Alert the student that you wish to discuss a concern – identify it with them and state that you want to allow some time to discuss it specifically.
2. **P**rivacy	This reduces interruptions and can generate a supportive environment for discussion. It also facilitates sensitive issues to surface. See the next box of reflection points.
3. **P**recision – an 'opening statement'	This can be especially helpful if the conversation is likely to be a sensitive or challenging one to address. It is worth rehearsing it to yourself beforehand: a simple, clear, non-judgemental single sentence articulating why you need to meet. Sometimes writing this first question or sentence down can be helpful for you to *fine-tune* it. Use objective criteria rather than comparisons to other people, for example.
4. **P**hones/distractions off	This reduces interruptions and can generate a supportive environment for discussion.
5. **P**lenty of time (more than you might expect . . .)	This is often a challenge in itself! You may need to enlist the support of a CTL or other manager to protect some time for the meeting.
6. **P**lan ahead – support for the student or yourself	Consider whether the meeting will affect the student's clinical work after the meeting. Might there be tears? Ought anyone else know that the meeting is scheduled? How will you both document what the meeting has covered and agreed?

life-experience do indicate that exposure to a wider world and broader range of people prior to becoming a student paramedic does help (Henderson 2012). Nonetheless, it is also acknowledged that age alone cannot pre-determine to what degree of such life experience has been garnered – the move to potentially younger students, for instance, is not inherently problematic!

The recent changes in paramedic education being situated in HEIs means that communication between practice and the *education provider* becomes critical; a degree of integration can be lost in the move away from *in-house* provision. Two points appear to be of singular importance:

1. The mentor's understanding of the lines of communication with the HEI.

2. The way that the students' practice placement documentation is intended to work in regards to communicating with the HEI.

Typically, students have personal tutors who are a first point of contact for points of concern and also for praising exceptional practice. The personal tutor should be identified in the student's practice placement document, or can be identified simply by contacting a member of the course/programme team: often there is a member of the course/programme team assigned as a *liaison* for each placement area. These initial points of contact will be able to escalate and prioritize responses as the situation requires. It is wise to document your own involvement here – email works well because it provides a timed and dated receipt, voice mail is less reliable in this regard. If there appear to be breaks or strong delays in the lines of communication, this may need to be brought to the course/programme leader's attention or raised at mentor update meetings, if these are available.

In case of these communication difficulties persisting, it is wise to alert the respective HEI, NHS and Ambulance Trust placement coordinators. There are frequently paramedics working in the HEI in a lecturer practitioner capacity who would be ideally suited to liaise between practice and HEI settings; they may be called upon to support students and staff in the mentoring process (Lavender 2013).

Students will have a portfolio or practice assessment document to evidence practice-based learning outcomes. These documents provide deliberate space to acknowledge both formative and summative points in their placement. The skills-specific elements are typically quite prescriptive in nature but there are other areas that support and feedback can be formally documented in. In Table 10.3 is a consideration of some of the mechanisms that are available to us to maintain a record of mentorship activity in these documents.

These practice assessment documents vary from institution to institution: you may well have other areas that serve you and the student well for recording discussions and development plans etc. In Table 10.4 are a few questions that may be useful in contemplating the document and our approaches to its use

The ideas in Table 10.4 are a very small fraction of the considerations and questions that can be asked of ourselves and our students. Mentoring students is uniquely rewarding. It unavoidably requires that we develop as practitioners ourselves – both in terms of our mentorship skills but also in terms of clinical practice very often, because students are the vanguard of new practice – we will, in fact, learn a huge amount from them.

This chapter has provided an insight into the preceptor and mentor role, the following case studies are provided in order that you think about some of the points mentioned throughout the chapter and possibly apply some strategies suggested to discuss if they may make your handling of certain situations easier and lead to a more satisfactory outcome for all concerned. Discuss your thoughts with colleagues and compare your thoughts.

Table 10.3 Maximizing the use of the student's practice assessment documentation

Element	Function	Comments
Self-assessment	Initiates discussion and forms the basis for *learning contracts* if they are used.	Can often be written in slightly negative terms - what they cannot do yet, etc. Encourage some acknowledgement of what they can already engage with, too.
Initial Interview	Contains the self-assessment and learning contract if used, and provides a sense of what the student hopes for from the placement.	Try and agree the date as early as possible. It may be worth indicating how you would like to use the document, for instance, if there is a troubling area that you will try and raise it early and agree an action plan together: this may *normalize* the process and make it appear less *punitive*.
Learning Contract	States the areas that the student wishes to focus on in terms of their own learning.	Students' learning is somewhat prescribed for them by way of the skills/learning outcomes expected in the practice assessment document.
Mid-Point Interview	*Looking back & looking forwards*: this is the point to adjust learning contracts as needed.	Try and agree the date as early as possible. This is an interview that is often missed but allows progress/challenges to be identified and action plans to be initiated/adapted. Critical feedback should not wait to the end-point interview. A good point to alert HEI if challenges are encountered
End-Point Interview	This is a reflective point and very useful to gauge progress both in terms of the learning contract, as well as elements that appear outside of it.	Try and agree the date as early as possible. If you are likely to see the student again – if they return to your practice area – you might use this as an element of the new learning contract/initial interview.
Action Plan	Details the steps needed to support & advance learning (can be knowledge/skills/attitudes).	Various models exist to support these, e.g. S.M.A.R.T: *Specific:* give unambiguous goals to achieve *Measurable & Mutual:* the goal is understood and agreed by both parties *Achievable:* within the student's capabilities *Realistic & Relevant:* the plan benefits the student in terms of their actual practice *Timebound:* an agreed time frame for review is agreed A good point to alert HEI when an action plan is agreed for a challenging issue.

Table 10.4 Considerations for mentorship documentation

Element	Consideration
Self- assessment	How might we need to support/encourage year 1 students in this?
	How can we address unrealistic self-assessment? When it is too elevated? When it is too critical?
Initial Interview	How can we plan for the initial interview? Is it the first time the student has met you as their mentor?
	Are they year 1, 2, 3? What are the differences between these students?
Learning Contract	Appropriate learning experiences for students ~ what is our role?
	Theory needed to support skills – how are they going to achieve this? How well do we need to know the course that they are undertaking?
Mid-Point Interview	Review self-assessment and invite a review of this so far.
	How is the learning contract or any action plan going? Review/renew/adapt.
End-Point Interview	Often a point to congratulate students on their successes and to help them look ahead to what is next on their course – possibly to help plan for that: can you help with that at all?
Action Plan	Is there a structure that you feel is appropriate, e.g. S.M.A.R.T?
	Is there anyone else that needs to know that this is in effect?

Case study 10.1

Adele is a very popular student whose enthusiasm is infectious and who seems to have been *adopted* by nearly all of your colleagues as *belonging* to your station; her time keeping, appearance and general attitude are excellent and many people have suggested that she be encouraged to apply for a post in the Trust as a Paramedic when she qualifies in a few months time as she fits in with the team really well.

As her mentor you have noted that her aseptic technique varies noticeably each time she is required to apply it and that each time there are fairly glaring errors that need to be addressed – it is something different every time and Adele is beginning to get frustrated with you and, you note, starting to shy away from situations that require her to use asepsis.

This is a mandatory skill in her skills practice assessment document and has been failed on her previous station and has been carried over to this placement. It did not surface in her initial interview between Adele and yourself.

How would you respond to the situation in terms of the following?

- knowledge
- skills
- attitudes

Who do you feel needs to be involved with any potential communication lines? Why?

What errors may have been made to date in supporting Adele, who is a year 3 student?

Case study 10.2

Charlie is 22 and a first year student on her second clinical placement with you. She has travelled round the world recently and been an Emergency Care Support Worker for the 2 years preceding this in a busy urban station. She is absolutely brimming with confidence – a life and soul of the party character – and seems to be very confident in practice; recently staff have commended her for her assertive response to a junior doctor's request that she tidies up after a clinical procedure in A&E.

Relatives of an elderly woman who is quite hard of hearing have mentioned to you that Charlie is *shouting* at their auntie and being very brusque with them.

When you ask Charlie about this, she is quite offended and states simply that at the University lecture on *care of the elderly* it was mentioned in a group discussion that it is necessary to speak clearly and loudly for those with hearing impairments – and that is all she is doing: she is just doing her job. She adds that she has met relatives like this before in her time as an Emergency Care Support Worker.

What do you think needs to be addressed in terms of the following?

- knowledge
- skills
- attitudes

Who do you feel needs to be involved with any potential communication lines? Why?

Having considered the role of mentor for students, it is important that the role of preceptor is explored. The remainder of this chapter will explore preceptorship as it relates to newly registered clinicians; it should be recognized that a similar process can also be used for new employees moving between Trusts.

Preceptorship

The value and importance of preceptorship is recognized in many policy drivers including *Framing the Contribution of Allied Health Professionals* (DH 2008a) and *High Quality Care for All: NHS Next Stage Review* (DH 2008b). *The Preceptorship Framework for Newly Registered Nurses, Midwives and Allied Health Professionals* was published by the Department of Health in 2010 (DH 2010). It developed from earlier work which initially focused on a review of Preceptorship for Nurses which was first introduced following the implementation of Project 2000 (DH 1999). Feedback suggested that the framework should be extended beyond nursing to include midwives and allied health professionals. The Department of Health engaged with stakeholders, the HCPC and NMC and reviewed models and approaches to Preceptorship with a specific focus on Scotland's 'Flying Start NHS', as this is a multi-professional preceptorship programme. Following this consultation, the revised document was launched (DH 2010).

The Preceptorship Framework for Nursing (DH 2009) provides clear principles for good preceptorship and practical and relevant information for employers to ensure equity of access for all newly registered practitioners. It is intended for use as a guide by NHS organizations who have responsibility for managing and developing the workforce and the launch of the framework document was supported by both the Chief Allied Health Professions Officer and the Chief Nursing Officer for England. To support the introduction of preceptorship programmes, dedicated Department of Health funding became available on a recurring basis in 2008/09 (DH 2009: 8)

Definitions of preceptorship

The Health and Care Professions Council do not formally define the term 'Preceptorship' but agreed as part of the Modernising Allied Health Careers Steering Group (2009) that preceptorship relates to enhancing practice. It is acknowledged that new registrants are safe and competent, but novice practitioners will continue to develop their competence as part of their career development. Preceptorship is about providing support and guidance to enable 'new registrants' to make the transition from student to accountable practitioner (NMC 2006). The period of preceptorship should provide the preceptee with the opportunity to practise in accordance with the HCPC standards for conduct, performance and ethics, whilst developing confidence in their competence as a 'Paramedic'.

Preceptorship is defined in many ways but the common factor in each is the central element of support. This is captured in the revised framework document as Preceptorship is defined as:

a period of structured transition for the newly registered practitioner during which he or she will be supported by a preceptor, to develop their confidence as an autonomous professional, refine skills, values and behaviours, and to continue on their journey of life-long learning.

(DH 2010: 11)

This definition and others reflect the fact that at the point of registration a paramedic is safe and competent as they must meet the required HCPC Standards of Proficiency and Standards of Education and Training to be eligible to apply for registration with the HCPC as a paramedic. Preceptorship is therefore not viewed as a way to meet any shortfall in pre-registration education but is recognized as a transition phase for newly registered practitioners when continuing their professional development. This provides an opportunity to build their confidence in decision-making and further develop competence for practice.

Having defined preceptorship, it is appropriate to consider what it is not. Preceptorship is not:

- intended to replace mandatory training programmes;
- intended to be a substitute for performance management processes;
- intended to replace regulatory body processes to deal with performance;
- an additional period in which another registrant takes responsibility and accountability for the newly registered practitioner's responsibilities and actions (i.e. it is not a further period of training);
- formal coaching (although coaching skills may be used by the preceptor to facilitate the learning of the newly registered practitioner);
- mentorship;
- statutory or clinical supervision;
- intended to replace induction to employment. (DH 2010: 12)

Preceptorship and accountability

From the moment a newly qualified paramedic registers with the HCPC, they become autonomous and accountable for their actions and clinical decisions. It is well documented that this transition period can result in high levels of anxiety for all newly qualified professionals and as far back as 1974 Kramer referred to the term *reality shock* to describe this period of transition for nurses (Kramer 1974).

The value and importance of preceptorship are recognized in the document *High Quality Workforce: NHS Next Stage Review* where it is acknowledged as a foundation period for practitioners at the start of their careers which supports them in their journey from novice to expert (DH 2008b).

Benner (2001) identifies the stages that an individual travels through before becoming an expert practitioner in their field of work. Benner introduced the concept that healthcare disciplines develop skills and understanding of patient care over time through a sound educational base which requires exposure to a multitude of experiences. Benner proposed that clinical experience is a prerequisite to becoming an expert practitioner and this is recognized in the student profile as they comment that their current role is ' [to] observe and support the senior clinician up to but not beyond my skill set as a student paramedic' (Clinician Profile: Student Paramedic). The student is recognizing their limitations but when asked to provide examples of the types of decisions made on a daily basis goes on to say:

> During my first two years of study I would say this question was nonapplicable as decisions were usually made without my input. However, during my third year after staff had gained trust and confidence in me, my ideas were sought more often.

This clearly demonstrates that the student has developed and is using prior knowledge and experience to inform current decision-making which is being recognized by the qualified member of staff supporting them in practice as well as the student. However, at the point of registration newly qualified paramedics could be still be described as novice practitioners as they have previously gained experience under the constant supervision of a qualified paramedic and mentor. Professional registration is a major leap in responsibility and accountability (Gopee 2011).

Self-evaluation exercise

Read Benner's (2001) – work *From Novice to Expert*, and consider where you are now in relation to your current role.

Purpose of preceptorship

It has been established that the purpose of preceptorship is to prepare newly qualified paramedics and other healthcare professionals for entry into the NHS workforce. This is in contrast to mentorship as mentors could be actively engaged in the assessment of students' practice to reach this point of registration. The HCPC strongly advocate the provision of preceptorship as a method for providing transitional role support from student to qualified practitioner status. It is recognized that this period of time following registration as a health care professional can be a challenging time and good support and guidance are essential. Newly registered paramedics and practitioners who manage the transition successfully are able to provide effective care more quickly, feel better about their role and more likely to remain in the profession. As a result, they make a greater contribution to patient care, but also ensure the benefits from the investment in their education is maximized (DH 2010: 4).

Preceptorship supports the policy drive to place quality at the heart of healthcare as confidence is created when patients see that individuals have the skills to do the job and the motivation to provide the level of care

(DH 2010). In addition, the Care Quality Commission requires providers to ensure workers are appropriately supported to enable them to deliver care and treatment safely and an effective preceptorship programme will contribute to achieving this.

The preceptor

A preceptor is a registered paramedic or health registered professional who has been given formal responsibility to support a newly qualified and registered paramedic/practitioner through a period of preceptorship. Clinical Leadership incorporates a number of elements, as discussed in previous chapters but one aspect is to develop others professionally to achieve their potential. This is recognized in the profile of the 'Paramedic Practitioner' job description as development and supervision of staff and students is one of the principal duties and responsibilities.

This is central to the support role of Preceptorship and leadership skills are acknowledged as one of the attributes of an effective preceptor as listed in Box 10.1.

Box 10.1 The attributes of an effective preceptor

- Giving constructive feedback.
- Setting goals and assessing competency.
- Facilitating problem solving.
- Active listening skills.
- Understanding, demonstrating and evidencing reflective practice ability in the working environment.
- Demonstrating good time management and leadership skills.
- Prioritizing care.
- Demonstrating appropriate clinical decision-making and evidence-based practice.
- Recognizing their own limitations and those of others.
- Knowing what resources are available and how to refer newly registered practitioners appropriately if additional support is required, for example, pastoral support or occupational health service.
- Being an effective and inspirational role model and demonstrating professional values, attitudes and behaviours.
- Demonstrating a clear understanding of the regulatory impact of the care that they deliver and the ability to pass on this knowledge.
- Providing a high standard of practice at all times.

Source: DH (2010: 17)

Preceptors are the key to the success of preceptorship programmes and should be appropriately prepared and supported to undertake the role. They should have 12 months post qualifying experience as a minimum and it is recommended that they complete a programme with a Higher Education Institution to develop their skills and knowledge of supporting students in practice (Gopee 2011).

Reflection: points to consider

What skills and qualities to you think you have that would make you a good preceptor to support students during their transition as a newly qualified registrant?

The preceptee

A preceptee is generally a newly qualified practitioner who has recently registered with the HCPC, but can be a qualified paramedic who is returning to practice following a long period of absence. Unlike many other professions, newly registered paramedics are often employed as lead clinicians from the outset of their career and consequently can lead a small team almost from the point of registration. Paramedics complete their programmes with the skills and knowledge they require to work as an independent practitioner, however, a period of preceptorship with an experienced paramedic will enable the new registrant to develop confidence in their decision-making skills as they function as a lead paramedic with the support of an experienced clinician.

Process

Preceptorship provides a structured process for the induction and development of staff employed in roles that require a significant level of knowledge and skills with some degree of autonomy. The content of a preceptorship programme should be planned in relation to the professional responsibilities of the newly qualified registrant and the needs of the employer. All learning undertaken during this period should be recorded in a manner that meets the requirements of the Key Skills Framework (KSF) appraisal process (or equivalent), any employer probationary requirements, continuing professional development and for paramedics returning to practice the revalidation requirements of the HCPC to avoid duplication of effort (DH 2010: 19). Two core components are identified as theoretical learning and guided reflection on practice. It is suggested that the period of support should be anything from 6–12 months and include 4–6 days of theoretical learning.

The College of Paramedics Paramedic Curriculum Guidance (COP 2013b) follows the suggested guidelines in the Preceptorship Framework (DH 2010) in relation to length of support and theoretical days. However, additional recommendations are made which focus specifically on the role of a paramedic as follows:

- During the first 6 months of practice following registration, newly qualified paramedics should not work as a lone responder.

- The first 150 hours post registration should include 'back-up' from an experienced paramedic with 12 months post registration experience.

- New registrants should not be on an active on call rota, unless responding as a team in exceptional circumstances.

- New registrants should not undertake supervision of a new member of emergency support staff or peers for at least 12 months following registration.

- 24-hour clinical telephone advice available to support decision-making skills.

Preceptorship in practice

North East Ambulance NHS Foundation Trust (NEAS) implemented Preceptorship in September 2012 following the guidance in the Preceptorship Framework document. Extensive consultation took place across the Trust and focus groups were undertaken with final year students near completion of the Foundation Degree Paramedic Science across the operational divisions to seek their views regarding the implementation of preceptorship. Although opinions were varied related to length of period for preceptorship, all staff viewed this as a positive way forward within the Trust. Commitment from all parties to successfully implement preceptorship is essential from the outset as introducing preceptorship as a support role is not without its challenges. It requires a *culture shift* within the ambulance service as previously newly qualified staff have learnt *on the job* and through experience. In addition, current staff who support students as mentors require education and updates related to the differences between the role of mentor and preceptor to enable the preceptee to develop their confidence and decision-making skills.

Preceptorship forms part of the Clinical Governance agenda to help employees achieve their full potential, while promoting patient safety through the provision of evidence-based high quality care. *Clinical Leadership in the Ambulance Services* (NHS 2009) defines clinical leadership as an 'expert clinician, involved in providing direct care, who influences others to improve the care they provide continuously' and NEAS have embedded preceptorship in their Leadership and Supervision Policy.

Preceptorship is available for all new registrants and the process includes the following:

- The period of preceptorship is one year.

- The first 8 weeks post qualification is rostered to work alongside an experienced paramedic to develop confidence in decision-making skills.

- The preceptee attends four study days throughout the year to reflect on practice and undertake critical incident analysis, providing an opportunity for sharing and learning with their peers.

- A review of progress and development is undertaken every three months to offer support to the preceptee.

- The six-month period includes a review for possibility of working as a lone responder.

- A portfolio is completed throughout the year to support personal development. This includes identification of individual learning needs through undertaking SWOT analysis and action plans.

- The portfolio forms part of a 20-credit module at level 6 within a local Higher Education Institution.

- Newly qualified practitioners have access to a 24-hour *on call clinician* to support their decision-making in practice.

An effective preceptorship programme will encourage and support individuals, while ensuring standards of proficiency are consistently achieved, thus reducing the risks and maintaining high levels of patient care and safety in the pre-hospital environment. On successful completion of preceptorship, it is anticipated that the registered practitioner will have become an effective, confident and fully autonomous registered individual who is able to deliver high quality care for patients, clients and service users. The expectation is that with effective support they will continue forward to become an independent and innovative leader as well as a role model for future generations (DH 2010: 21).

Conclusion

In conclusion, this chapter has outlined the key differences between the support roles of mentorship and preceptorship and discussed how they can be utilized effectively to support learning in practice. Both roles are exceptionally important, both to the individual students and to the organization as a whole and form part of the Clinical Governance agenda to help employees achieve their full potential, while promoting patient safety through the provision of evidence-based high quality care.

The roles are often viewed as additional responsibility when in reality a mentor/preceptor has the potential to *make or break* the students' practice experience within an organization. The chapter has explained the origins of both roles, future opportunities and has explored some key points in relation to becoming a successful mentor/preceptor. There are numerous points on which you are encouraged to reflect and some case studies which will generate thought, discussion and have the potential for establishing new ways of working.

Chapter key points

- Both mentorship and preceptorship have strong research-based and policy-driven roots.

- Mentorship and preceptorship are important and valuable roles within an organization.

- There are clearly defined roles for both mentor and preceptor and each offer valuable support for learning in practice.

- All newly registered paramedics should have a structured period of preceptorship in line with the CoP Framework recommendations.

- Both roles can be challenging, but there are recommended strategies available to make the process structured and beneficial to both parties.

- The changing demographics of student paramedics' education bring some unique challenges to the paramedic profession.

References and suggested reading

Armitage, E. (2011) Role of paramedic mentors in an evolving profession, *Journal of Paramedic Practice*, 2(1): 26–31.

Armstrong, N. (2010) Clinical mentors' influence on student midwives' clinical practice, *British Journal of Midwifery*, 18(2): 114–23.

Benner, P. (2001) *From Novice to Expert: Excellence and Power in Clinical Nursing Practice*. London: Prentice Hall.

Bower, J.L., Wainright, J.M., Cropley, M. and Willaims, K.L. (2012) *Physical Fitness, Sleep Hygiene and Work Related Well Being Markers in Paramedics*. Surrey: University of Surrey.

Brown, L., Douglas, V., Garrity, J. and Shepard, C.K. (2012) What influences mentors to pass or fail students? *Nursing Management*, 19(5): 16–21.

Cassidy, S. (2009) Interpretation of competence in student assessment, *Nursing Standard*, 23(18): 39–46.

College of Paramedics (2008) *Paramedic Curriculum Guidance and Competence Framework*. Derby: College of Paramedics.

College of Paramedics (2013a) *Paramedic Curriculum Guidance*, 3rd edn. Bridgwater: College of Paramedics.

College of Paramedics (2013b) *Forum for Higher Education in Paramedic Science*. Minutes: 17.04.2013.

Council of Deans of Health (2009) Report from the preceptorship workshops retreat, Bristol, 27 May 2009 (unpublished).

Department of Health (1999) *Making a Difference: Strengthening the Nursing, Midwifery and Health Visiting Contribution to Health and Healthcare*. London: Department of Health.

Department of Health (2008a) *Framing the Contribution of Allied Health Professionals: Delivering High-Quality Healthcare*. London: Department of Health.

Department of Health (2008b) *High Quality Care for All: NHS Next Stage Review Final Report*. CM 7432. London: Department of Health.

Department of Health (2009) *Preceptorship Framework for Nursing.* London: Department of Health. Available at: http://webarchive.nationalarchives.gov.uk/+/ www.dh.gov.uk/prod_consum_dh/groups/dh_digitalassets/@dh/@en/@abous/ documents/digitalasset/dh_109794.pdf (accessed 20 August 2013).

Department of Health (2010) *Preceptorship Framework for Newly Registered Nurses, Midwives and Allied Health Professionals.* London: Department of Health.

Donaghy, J. (2011) The student experience of university paramedic education/training – from classroom learning to situational understanding. In preparation for the award of Professional Doctorate in Education (EdD) University of Hertfordshire (unpublished).

Donaldson, J.H. and Carter, D. (2005) The value of role modelling: perceptions of undergraduate and diploma nursing (adult) students, *Nurse Education in Practice,* 5: 353–9.

Davies, D. (2013) Social media: the good, the bad and the ugly, *Journal of Paramedic Practice,* 5(5): 294–5.

Duffy, K. (2003) *Failing Students: A Qualitative Study of Factors that Influence the Decisions Regarding Assessment of Students' Competence in Practice.* Available at: http:// www.nmc-uk.org/Documents?Archived%20Publications/1Research%20papers/ Kathleen_Duffy_Failing_Students2003.pdf (accessed 2 March 2013).

Eva, K.W., Rosenfeld, J., Reiter, H.I. and Norman, G.R. (2004) An admissions OSCE: the multiple mini-interview, *Medical Education,* 38: 314–26.

Gopee, N. (2011) *Mentoring and Supervision in Healthcare,* 2nd edn. London: Sage.

Health and Care Professions Council (2012a) *Standards for Education and Training.* London: HCPC.

Health and Care Professions Council (2012b) *Your Guide to Our Standards for Continuing Professional Development.* London: HCPC.

Health and Care Professions Council (2012c) *Guidance on Conduct and Ethics for Students.* London: HCPC.

Health and Care Professions Council (2012d) *Standards of Proficiency: Paramedics.* London: HCPC.

Health and Care Professions Council (2013a) *Register of Approved Programmes.* Available at:http://www.hpc-uk.org/education/programmes/register/index.asp?intStartRow=1 &EducationProviderID=all&StudyLevel=all&ProfessionID=10&PostRegistrationID= &ModeOfStudyID=all&RegionID=17,%2020,%207,%2015,%2016,%2013,%2014,%2018, %2019,%209,%208,%2010#educationSearchResults (accessed 1 May 2013).

Health and Care Professions Council (2013b) *Focus on Standards: Social Networking Sites.* Available at: http://www.hcpc-uk.org/Assets/documents/100035B7Social_ media_guidance.pdf (accessed 1 June 2013).

Health and Safety Executive (2012) *Musculoskeletal Disorders.* Available at: http:// www.hse.gov.uk/statistics/causdis/musculoskeletal/msd.pdf (accessed 13 May 2013).

Health and Safety Executive (2013) *Stress and Psychological Disorders.* Available at: http://www.hse.gov.uk/statistics/causdis/stress/stress.pdf (accessed 13 May 2013).

Health and Social Care Information Centre (2013) *Sickness Absence Rates in the NHS: October–December 2012.* Available at: https://catalogue.ic.nhs.uk/publications/ workforce/sickness/sick-abse-rate-nhs-oct-dec-2012/sick-abse-rate-nhs-oct-dec-2012-rep.pdf (accessed 13 May 2013).

Hegg-Deloye, S., Brassard, P., Jauvin, N., Prairie, J., Larouche, D., Poirier, P., Tremblay, A. and Corbeil, P. (2014) Current state of knowledge of post-traumatic stress, sleeping problems, obesity and cardiovascular disease in paramedics. *Emergency Medicine Journal,* 31(3): 242–70.

Henderson, T. (2012) Influence of life experience on undergraduate paramedic students' placements, *Journal of Paramedic Practice,* 4(10): 585–92.

Jones, A., Slater, J. and Griffiths, P. (2010) *The First Year Experiences of Paramedic Students in Higher Education.* The Higher Education Academy: Health Sciences and Practice. [Online] Available at: http://www.heacademy.ac.uk/assets/documents/subjects/health/aledjones[1].jpg. (accessed 1 March 2013).

Jones, P., Comber, J. and Conboy, A. (2012) The art and science of mentorship in action, *Journal of Paramedic Practice* 4(8): 474–9.

King, L.M., Jackson, M.T., Gallagher, A., Wainwright, P., and Lindsay, J. (2009) Towards a model of the expert practice educator – interpreting multi-professional perspectives in the literature, *Learning in Health and Social Care*, 8(2): 135–44.

Kramer, M. (1974) *Why Nurses Leave Nursing.* London: Mosby.

Lavender, D. (2013) Is the role of the paramedic lecturer practitioner fit for purpose? *Journal of Paramedic Practice*, 5(6): 326–30.

Lemay, J.F., Lockyer, J.M., Collin, V.T. and Brownell, A.K.W. (2007) Assessment of non-cognitive traits through the admissions multiple mini-interview, *Medical Education*, 1: 573–9.

Mildenhall, J. (2012a) Occupational stress, paramedic informal coping strategies: a review of the literature, *Journal of Paramedic Practice*, 4(6): 318–28.

Mildenhall, J. (2012b) Occupational cup of tea and a chat? Get the kettle on.... *Journal of Paramedic Practice*, 4(4): 191.

NHS Ambulance Chief Executive Group (2009) *Report of the National Steering Group on Clinical Leadership in the Ambulance Service.* London: NHS.

Nursing and Midwifery Council (2006a) *Preceptorship Guidelines.* Available at: http://www.google.com/search?sitesearch=&q=Nursing+and+Midwifery+Council+preceptorship+2006 (accessed 18 August 2013).

Nursing and Midwifery Council (2006b) *Standards to Support Learning and Assessment in Practice: NMC Standards for Mentors, Practice Teachers and Teachers.* London: NMC.

Pointer, J.E. (2001) Experience and mentoring requirements for competence in new/inexperienced paramedics. *Pre-hospital Emergency Care*, 5(4): 379–83.

Ryan, L. and Halliwell, D. (2012) Paramedic decision making: how is it done? *Journal of Paramedic Practice*, 4(6): 343–51.

Sibson, L. and Mursell, I. (2010a) Mentorship for paramedic practice: are we there yet? *Journal of Paramedic Practice* 2(5): 206–9.

Sibson, L. and Mursell, I. (2010b) Mentorship for paramedic practice: bridging the gap, *Journal of Paramedic Practice*, 2(6): 270–4.

Skingley, A., Arnott, J., Greaves, J. and Nabb, J. (2007) Supporting practice teachers to identify failing students, *British Journal of Community Nursing*, 12(1): 28–32.

Van der Gaag, A. and Donaghy, J. (2013) Paramedics and professionalism: looking back and looking forwards, *Journal of Paramedic Practice*, 5(1): 8–10.

Williams, A. (2012) Emotion work in paramedic practice: the implications for nurse educators, *Nurse Education Today*, 32: 368–72.

Williams, A. (2013) The strategies used to deal with emotion work in student paramedic practice, *Nurse Education in Practice*, 13: 207–12.

Woollard, M. (2009) Professionalism in UK paramedic practice, *Journal of Emergency Primary Health Care*, 7(4): 1–6.

Useful website

http://www.flyingstartengland.nhs.uk/preceptors.htm.

Conclusion

Amanda Blaber and Graham Harris

We are in challenging times for the NHS in England. The importance of clinical leadership has vacillated on and off the agenda for a number of years, but at no time in the past has it been so important that NHS Trusts need to rely on the leaders within their workforce and support them to lead from within their organization. We believe this is the only way NHS Trusts will be able to achieve all that the government is asking of them.

The timely publication of this book should assist students and registered paramedics to explore the array of subjects that are inextricably linked to clinical leadership. The paramedic profiles provide some insight into the role of clinical leadership that exists on a day-to-day basis for some staff. It is worth noting that leadership responsibilities do not appear to extend past the point of patient care delivery for many clinicians. The new era of *leadership* in the NHS may require all staff to take more organizational responsibility in the future.

As with any academic subject area, opinions vary, debates ensue and differences remain. This book should serve as a *starting point* for your reading and investigation. Through your reading you will develop your own beliefs and theories about how clinical leadership works best for you as an individual; for your role; the organization and ultimately for the patient. As the government has made clear with their response to the Francis Report, Patients *First and Foremost* (DH 2013), the patient experience will be central to NHS decision-making for the foreseeable future. The people who have a direct effect on the patient experience are frontline staff. It is, therefore, vital that clinical leaders are developed, supported and listened to, as they will be a vital component of the future success of the NHS. In response to the Francis Inquiry recommendations, the NHS Leadership Academy have released a Healthcare Leadership Model (2013), stating that it is not 'set in stone' and will continue developing and being updated so it remains relevant to staff for a longer period of time.

We end where we started with the introduction to this book, with the findings of the Francis Report (Mid Staffordshire NHS Foundation Trust Public Inquiry 2013). The Report recognized that the recommendations made would not be achieved in a matter of weeks, rather it could take months or years. The Report is clear in its assertion that clinical leadership is central to the achievement of the recommendations.

References

Department of Health (2013) *Patients First and Foremost. The Initial Government Response to the Report of the Mid Staffordshire NHS Foundation Trust Public Inquiry.* London: The Stationery Office.

Mid Staffordshire NHS Foundation Trust Public Inquiry (2013) *Report of the Mid Staffordshire NHS Foundation Trust Public Inquiry.* Executive Summary. Chaired by Robert Francis QC. London: The Stationery Office.

NHS Leadership Academy (2013) *Healthcare Leadership Model: The Nine Dimensions of Leadership Behaviour.* Version 1.0 NHS Leadership Academy. Leeds. Available at: www.leadershipacademy.nhs.uk/leadershipmodel (accessed 26 November 2013).

Index

Locators shown in *italics* refer to figures, tables, boxes and case studies.